W9-CPQ-607

THE NATURAL WAY

TO

HEALTHFUL SLEEP

THE NATURAL WAY TO
HEALTHFUL SLEEP

by **CHARLES P. KELLY**

with an introduction by
MAURICE E. LINDEN, M.D.
Assistant Professor of Psychiatry
University of Pennsylvania
School of Medicine

DARTON, LONGMAN & TODD   LONDON

Darton, Longman & Todd Ltd.,
29a Gloucester Road,
London, S.W.7.

© 1961 by Charles P. Kelly
First edition published 1961
This edition published 1962

Acknowledgments

Much of the material in this book has come from the author's own original experiments. Other material has been gathered over a period of years from many different sources. It is not possible to give credit to all these sources, though a number of the more important ones are mentioned at appropriate places in the text. For their prompt and careful replies to his inquiries, the author would like to express his appreciation to Nathaniel Kleitman, H. M. Johnson, W. O. Fenn, Gudmund Magnussen, Buckminster Fuller, A. G. Bills, James Bender and also, if he were still living, to W. B. Cannon. For their assistance and friendly interest over the years while basic material for the book was being gathered the author is deeply grateful to Doctor John L. Evers, zoologist, and Professor George H. Satterfield, physiological chemist, both of the North Carolina State College faculty, and he is greatly indebted to Mrs. Katherine Edsall of the North Carolina State College library for her interested and efficient aid in securing material from other libraries. Thanks are due from the author to a number of libraries for courtesies shown him when he was consulting their files. He especially appreciates the aid received from the National Library of Medicine in Washington, the medical library of Duke University, and the general and specialized libraries of North Carolina State College, their very competent services having been used by him almost continuously for a number of years past. However, the author is most indebted to his son, Doctor William E. Kelly, a psychiatrist on the faculty of Jefferson Medical College in Philadelphia, who read the entire manuscript and suggested a number of additions and revisions which are included in this final version.

To the doctor
who was first to recognize fully the
purpose and possibilities of this book,
and who gave so unstintingly of his time
to aid in their realization.

"A hypothesis which will be adequate to the task of explaining the phenomenon of sleep has, so far, not yet been propounded. Freud held out the theory of rhythmic return to inter-uterine Nirvana. Von Economo assumed that sleep supervenes upon a lack of incoming stimuli. The supposition of chemical substances of a catabolic kind, or of endocrine substances, circulating in the cerebrospinal fluid, is a well-known theory. And, more recently, a great deal of research work has been carried out with the view of discovering both the existence of a sleep center and the mechanism of its activation. Clinico-pathological studies, however, have failed to reach unanimity as to the location of such a center."

—Dr. William A. O'Connor, in The Practitioner

"It is truly strange that we know almost nothing of the mechanism by which sleep is produced. We spend almost a third of our lives asleep, and the physiology of this condition is less understood than is that of digestion or respiration. Further, the fact that we know little or nothing of the background of this state of being doesn't seem to occur to the minds of persons who spend their lives in physiological research."

—Dr. Foster Kennedy, in the New York State
Journal of Medicine

Introduction

My interest in this book stems from a variety of noteworthy factors. First, it happens that one of my very dear social and professional friends is the author's physician son referred to in the text. Together we have given much thought to the factual detail that is both educational to the reader and substantiating to the viewpoint presented. We have both studied the manuscript with care, and have made recommendations where appropriate.

It is an understatement to say that we are intrigued by the author's sleep-inducing method and its effectiveness.

Second, one of my professional avocations is that of gerontologist—student of aging. For over a decade I have been calling attention to the great intellectual potentials that too often lie dormant and untapped in the minds of people of the very advanced ages. In author Charles Kelly, a man nearing 90, we find just the kind of application of mental effort we can most heartily endorse. It is safe to say he is old in years only. There is every evidence of a continuing intellectual and psychological vigor in the author who has taken many years of arduous trial and methodical investigation to arrive at his point of view. The spontaneity, dedication, critical appraisal, and spirit of inquiry that are the very nature of the ever young creative scholar are very much in evidence in this book's contents.

Third, my work in the field of Public Mental Health has long led to searches for natural and economical means of maintaining emotional well-being and preventing psychological ill health. Certainly restful sleep must be regarded as an important resource for mental well-being. Not only is sleep one of nature's means of replenishing energy systems and aiding in general repair and healing processes ("sleep that knits up the ravell'd sleave of care"), but it is also an opportunity for problem-solving. Modern legend has it that in 1865 the German chemist Friedrich Kekulé—long troubled by the puzzle of the benzene molecule (C_6H_6)—worked out the problem in a dream while dozing. His dream of snakes and atoms, one snake whirling with its tail in its mouth, led to the concept of the benzene ring. People undergoing psychotherapy or psychoanalysis often long for sleep for the essential purpose of having a dream which hopefully may aid in solving some of the deeper psychological problems under consideration.

In the latter part of the nineteenth century and the early part of this one, sleep, rest and copious good food were prescribed for "nervous breakdowns." Many emotionally disturbed people spontaneously seek sleep as repose, respite from worry, and escape from the demands of reality. People who get along on a minimum of nocturnal sleep are often found to be capable of "cat napping" during the day, as was the case with Thomas A. Edison. Many working people enjoy separating the working day from the leisurely evening by drawing a transitional curtain of sleep.

The search for sleep is a problem probably as old as mankind. The earliest recorded history in practically every human culture has something to say about some individual desperately seeking sleep and the method whereby he found it. Magical potions, drugs, herbs, secret incantations and divine favor were among the agencies credited with aiding sleep. But all accounts had one thing in common—sleep did not always come easily and naturally when desired.

The same problem is true of today's world and may in fact be intensified by the complexity, pace and pressures of modern living. Judging from medical experience and the flourishing drugstore sales of sedatives and tranquilizers, millions of people must be plagued by the constant need to relax after a hectic day of living and the need to get rest and renewed energies with which to face hectic days to follow. For this reason today any book on sleep is likely to be sought and read by millions.

The present volume, however, is not just another book on sleep. *This is an original and new approach to the quest for sleep.* The heart of this method of obtaining sleep is found in the special breathing program the author describes and explains in detail. To be sure, some of the already validated measures aiding sleep are also utilized in this method. But the essence of author Kelly's original sleep-inducing regimen is controlled breathing.

It is not unusual in the ordinary course of human events for man's knowledge in a particular field to reach a plateau and remain there for a relatively long period. Then a sudden new understanding sends man's knowledge to a higher level. This is a "breakthrough." It is entirely conceivable that this book represents such an advance, for in all truth little else that is new has been added for several decades to our methods of obtaining sleep. Coué's autosuggestion and Jacobson's muscle relaxation methods practically sum up the list.

Recent advances in medically induced sleep have occurred, but everyone would agree that such artificial methods possessing some degree of potential hazard are still far from a satisfactory answer. A mode of inducing sleep such as author Kelly's is not only quick, easy and safe, but may well prove to be a scientific breakthrough which will simultaneously help master the age-old problem of sleep and be a contribution to man's knowledge, carrying us to a new plateau.

Two questions that inevitably arise in evaluating this method are: first, how effective is it? and second, how does it work? The first question is far more easily answered than the second.

This sleep-inducing method does work. It worked for the author, who, accidentally, came upon the method while seeking relief earlier in his life from his own problem of insomnia. It has worked for others who have learned of the method from the author. I have tried the method and have found it effective. Its use requires that it be clearly understood and conscientiously applied. The question of effectiveness can be answered in the affirmative.

The question of how the method works is at present not readily answered. Author Kelly has sought the answers to this question for more than fifteen years in a painstaking and careful project of research that has carried him to most of the leading scientific libraries in the country. It has led to correspondence with outstanding physiologists and medical specialists in inhalation physiology. As a result, the author has come to a theoretical explanation of how his method works, viz.: that the induced sleep is due to the increase in carbon dioxide content of the body brought about by controlled breathing.

Some individuals would say that this is too simple an answer. I would be inclined to agree with them, but until we understand the more profound biochemical complexities of the method, the simple answer seems satisfactory.

Some people might say that if an increase in carbon dioxide bodily concentration is all that is needed to obtain sleep, why not take a few whiffs of carbon dioxide on retiring at night? Or better yet, why not just take some baking soda, which, in the stomach, will quickly release carbon dioxide that is rapidly absorbed by the body.

A clear understanding of the basic principles of inhalation physiology would forestall such questions. In the case of inhaling carbon dioxide (CO_2), we know that CO_2 stimulates respiration. Increased and accelerated lung action would soon drive off the excess CO_2 and we would be right back where we started. The same ultimate effect would result from the taking of bicarbonate of (baking) soda, except that there is an added danger here of over-alkalinizing the body and producing generalized muscle tension. The author's method apparently increases the carbon dioxide content of the body by controlled, disciplined, and minimal breathing, which enables the body to build up its own natural supply of carbon dioxide. In this way the physiological state is set for natural sleep. The body automatically continues this minimal breathing and thus maintains the increased CO_2 concentration that is well known always to accompany sleep.

Further studies, clinical and scientific investigation are needed to validate the author's theory of operation of the method. Such studies are already well along in planning stages in one medical research laboratory in the country, having been stimulated by a reading of the manuscript by a leading physiologist prior to its publication. It may be expected that other related studies will follow.

Even without further laboratory confirmation, it may be said that the controlled breathing method of inducing sleep appears to be entirely consistent with the presently known principles of inhalation physiology. *Whatever future research discovers, the simple fact remains that this method of obtaining sleep works and is safe and wholesome.*

As an easily mastered method, it merits publication for use by the millions of sufferers of sleeplessness, or even for those who would like to learn the trick of cat napping at odd hours during the day.

So, as a student of human nature, physician to the ill, servant to the weary, and seeker after knowledge, I commend this book to the unrested and the rested—to the former as a means to comfort —to the latter as an exciting adventure in and satisfier of curiosity about the mastery of one of nature's most elusive yet basic needs— sleep.

MAURICE E. LINDEN, M.D.
Director, Division of Mental Health
Public Health Services
Dept. of Public Health, Philadel-
    phia, Pa.

and

Assistant Professor of Psychiatry
University of Pennsylvania School
    of Medicine
Philadelphia, Pa.

Contents

Appendix A

Appendix B

Appendix C

Appendix C

How an Amazing Gas Does So Many Things for Us   295

THE NATURAL WAY

TO

HEALTHFUL SLEEP

1. How to recapture
natural sleep

You Can Sleep at Will

Here, at last, is a real advance in the search for sleep.

This book will show you how, by a few simple exercises which you can practice in bed—basically nothing more complicated than taking a few controlled breaths, and following a few other equally simple directions—you can make yourself the master of the sleep-producing processes of your own body.

If you follow these suggestions, you won't need tranquilizers. You can throw away your sleeping pills.

Your body actually produces its own tranquilizer. That tranquilizer and sleep-producer is the gas, carbon dioxide. What carbon dioxide is and means to the body will be explained later. But at this point it is enough to say that when this gas increases sufficiently in your system sleep comes over you.

This book will show you how you can assist and control the production of this sleep-producing element in your own body, voluntarily, increasing the amount at will so that you can go to sleep when you want to sleep and when you are most worried and most need sleep.

Carbon dioxide is thrown off by each of us in the breath we exhale. By the proper control of your breathing when you put your head on your pillow you can woo and win sleep almost immediately.

This carbon dioxide is always available to you. And for speed of results, convenience in use, freedom from harmful effects, restfulness of sleep, and absence of hangover, this substance is unequalled by any known drug. Further, it requires no previous preparation, needs no special equipment, involves no expense and develops no intolerance or addiction.

Unnatural Sleep Not As Good As Natural Sleep

If you consult your physician for relief of insomnia and he is convinced that you are unable to get adequate sleep, he will first search for the cause of the insomnia, endeavoring to determine whether it is organic, that is, due to disease, or whether it is due to a psychological condition. He will probably give advice as to favorable conditions for sleep. He may discuss such aids as healthy exercise and correct evening diet, as well as the elements of proper mental hygiene which facilitate relaxation and sleep. But all too often the physician's best advice does not solve the problem and he is forced to rely for treatment upon hypnotic drugs such as the barbiturates, even though he knows in some cases these drugs are capable of causing a stubborn and dangerous drug habit. Unfortunately, many patients are tempted to continue using drugs and may discover, when it is too late, they are victims of a habit which, even with special treatment, is very hard to break.

Only two methods have ever been used successfully to produce sleep. One is to relieve the brain of stimuli coming from the five senses. Popular books and magazine articles on sleep follow this method, often using mysterious "tricks" and "sleep rituals," without any attempt to explain how they work. When the tendency to wakefulness is only slight, these devices may limit the flow of nerve impulses to the brain sufficiently to bring sleep. But nerve impulses bring reports from both outside and inside the body, many coming from various parts of the brain itself. And these impulses are of so many types and come from so many sources that adequate control of them is extremely difficult. Thus, when doctors must make sure of the patients' sleep they do not depend upon these control devices.

Even if nerve impulses coming to the brain could be controlled, this would still be only a negative procedure, just a clearing of the road for sleep. It offers no positive force to bring sleep. Sufferers from insomnia find that efforts to relax the muscles, exclusion of light and noise, and schemes for quieting the mind fail to give them relief. Such devices do not give the necessary final positive push into slumberland.

In laboratory experiments on animals sleep has been produced by surgical incisions in the brain and also by application of electrical currents. No practical use in ordinary sleep production has been found for these procedures. But to produce a direct effect upon the brain by means of drugs is both easy and practical. These drugs are simply chemicals which enter the blood stream and so change the chemistry of the brain. They are sometimes given by hypodermic injection, but swallowing a pill or powder is equally effective, for it quickly reaches the blood stream through the stomach. The ease, convenience, and positive effect of the chemical method of inducing sleep makes it a temptation to both doctor and patient, leading to the present enormous use of sleeping pills. Unfortunately, extensive research has not yet discovered a completely safe drug that will produce natural sleep. The sleep produced is unnatural, and continued use of the drug is unsafe.

Your Sleep-producing Hormone and Kety's Demonstration

In the absence of other effective means of securing natural sleep, and with the need for such a means being so evident and so widespread, it is somewhat surprising that the presence in our own bodies of a hormone-like substance ideally suited to fill the need seems to have been almost completely overlooked. It is not merely that we have not learned to use this potent product of the body. We are not even aware that we have such a priceless endowment. By the millions we pay our money for drugs that not only are potentially dangerous but are not nearly as well suited to our needs as this natural product which we have in our own bodies. This long-neglected but potent product is the once unappreciated but now widely utilized gas, carbon dioxide, which constantly escapes from our lungs in our breath.

The important part which carbon dioxide plays in the coming of sleep was strikingly demonstrated, and that somewhat unexpectedly, in a recent investigation carried out by Dr. Seymour Kety and his associates at the University of Pennsylvania, reported in the Journal of Clinical Investigation for July, 1955. Exact measurements were made of a number of physiological conditions in the brain, both during and preceding sleep. Fifty complete sets of measurements were made on young men who, being kept awake beyond their bedtime, were quite sleepy when the measurements began. Yet of the fifty tests the electroencephalograph showed that only six men were able to fall into sound sleep. This, of course, raised the question whether it was some difference in the brain condition of these six men that made it possible for them to pass into the unconsciousness of sleep while the others could not. A detailed examination was made of all the records of all the men both before and during sleep in an effort to find out what this difference might have been. Only one difference could be found. The six men who went to sleep had more carbon dioxide in their blood than the others, and this condition distinguished the six who slept from all the others not only during sleep but also in the period preceding sleep. While the measurements taken in this experiment did not indicate by what physiological process carbon dioxide promoted sleep, they did indicate strongly the important or even essential part which it plays in the approach of natural sleep.

This increase of carbon dioxide was evidently due to a decrease of breathing, and was therefore termed by the doctors a "respiratory acidosis." It has long been known that the carbon dioxide content of the blood is increased during sleep, and it is well known that all sleep-producing drugs, in addition to dulling the brain, also tend to reduce breathing and in this way produce a certain degree of "respiratory acidosis," more carbon dioxide in the blood. However, until Dr. Kety's experiment, it seems that little consideration had been given to the possibility that this increase of carbon dioxide might play an important part in bringing sleep. Now the doctors say in reporting their experiment that their findings have raised the question whether it is possible for a person to go to sleep without the aid of this "respiratory acidosis."

The point that interests us in connection with this experiment is that we can when we wish take voluntary control of our breathing and thus make purposeful use of "respiratory acidosis." No doubt the normal person whose body is tired and whose mind is at rest automatically and unconsciously reduces his breathing as he composes himself for sleep, thus bringing about the increase of carbon dioxide in his blood which the doctors suggest is probably necessary as a preparation for sleep. But when the body is tense or the mind excited, breathing is likely to be increased rather than reduced, thus washing carbon dioxide out of the blood and causing increased alkalinity instead of acidosis. Undoubtedly it is the absence of this normal respiratory acidosis which accounts for much insomnia. What probably happened in this experiment was that six of the men were so little affected by the circumstances of the test and the annoyance of the various instruments attached to them that they composed themselves and prepared for sleep in their customary manner, including a reduction of breathing, while all the others were so excited that they breathed normally or even increased their breathing. Consequently they not only prevented any increase of the carbon dioxide in their blood but even decreased it below its normal amount. And without this "respiratory acidosis" they could not go to sleep, even though they were very sleepy.

It is of interest to note that the author knew nothing of Dr. Kety's experiment until the report of it was published, while both the author and a few of his friends had already been using voluntarily produced respiratory acidosis as an aid to sleep for more than eight years previously. Yet the experiment could hardly have offered stronger support for the breathing procedures which had been developed if it had been deliberately planned for this purpose.

Although science has failed to propose any practical application for this information, the author of this book, after months of frightened groping for relief from exhausting insomnia, has had his health changed by the fortunate discovery of his unique system of voluntarily controlled breathing which induces sleep pleasantly and naturally, often within a few minutes.

The author's system is based on a breathing pattern which results in respiratory acidosis or retention of carbon dioxide, just as was found by the doctors in Pennsylvania, and it is entirely consistent with the best scientific knowledge thus far available on the subject.

Summary: Sleep Command Is Wholly Yours

The purpose of this book is to give the reader conscious command of the increase of carbon dioxide in the blood, and instead of leaving it to the good fortune of unconscious automatic production, to make it a voluntary and purposeful act. For bringing this potent aid to sleep under conscious control, tested procedures are fully described which will enable anyone to put this highly effective aid into use whenever it is needed for the purpose of overcoming wakefulness. For still greater effectiveness, these procedures have been arranged in such a way as to bring to bear at the same time other natural sleep-inducing resources of the body and the mind, the result being a forceful combination which gives an assured command of sleep under all ordinary conditions.

It is not the author's intention to amuse or entertain the reader, or merely to give information. His aim is to afford training, to give skill, to teach an accomplishment—a skill or accomplishment which will enable its possessor to approach every undertaking, whether work or play, in a fresh, rested, and fit condition, thus making a vast difference in every aspect of life. No space has been given to a repetition of tales and superstitions concerning sleep, or to the many entertaining though ineffectual systems for bringing sleep that have been suggested in the past. Scientific research, unfortunately, has so far suggested little beyond these folk stories. But the author brings a proved and practical method to assist the reader in achieving sleep easily, safely, and promptly.

Under appropriate chapter headings will be found sensible and dependable information on a number of subjects which are of practical interest in connection with sleep, such as ventilation of the bedroom, midday naps, dreams, snoring, fatigue, relaxation, relation of the eyes to sleep, control of external disturbances, and various other significant topics.

One chapter discusses in some detail the use of the body's own production of carbon dioxide as an aid to sleep.

In the appendix will be found brief sketches of some of the myriad other uses of this remarkable gas.

2. Why this natural method of inducing sleep is harmless, drugged sleep dangerous

Pills No Permanent Answer to Insomnia

A brief sketch of the events which led me to write this book may help the reader to a clear grasp of the new procedures it proposes for bringing safe and healthful sleep.

Upon again taking charge of my classes at North Carolina State College following a period of illness, I found myself lying awake most of the night, though my need for rest and recuperation demanded that I should be sleeping soundly. This was something new to me. I had never before had any trouble going to sleep promptly and sleeping soundly. Loss of sleep soon began to cut into the meager reserve of strength which I had built up during my recovery, and I realized that eventually I would be forced to drop my work again, this time probably permanently.

I went back to my doctor who had treated my sickness and he gave me a prescription for sleeping powders. He assured me that the powders contained no "dope," which probably meant that they consisted of one or more barbiturates but did not contain opiates. I was to take a powder about an hour before bedtime, whenever it seemed likely I would not be able to sleep without it.

In my weakened and nervous condition these instructions simply meant that I would be taking a powder every night, probably for an indefinite period. I realized, as I thought it over, that under such conditions there was serious danger of my becoming permanently dependent on the powders for sleep, with the final effect very likely being complete loss of health, both physical and mental. This brought me face to face with a frightening choice. I must, it seemed, break down immediately from loss of sleep or go to pieces eventually from the use of sleeping powders.

As I turned over in my mind these grim alternatives I found a sort of desperate faith or conviction building up within me that there must be some kind of procedure which would bring sleep without the use of brain-paralyzing drugs, and with this conviction came a belief that by persistent search such a procedure could be found. I knew so little about the physiology of sleep that I was obliged, as Boss Kettering says, quoting Edison, "to start with the facts, the problem, not with the preconceptions." So, driven by the urgency of my situation, I began my search.

Breathe Your Way to Drowsiness

The first natural condition that occurred to me as probably offering aid was fatigue, which is popularly credited with an almost magic ability to bring sleep. But here I was confronted with the problem of finding a means of producing fatigue that was suited to my weakened condition. Games or gymnasium work were beyond my strength. Even a short walk brought something more akin to exhaustion than fatigue. I recalled that many years ago I had seen an outline of breathing exercises which its advocates claimed was more beneficial than calisthenics or setting-up exercises, better even than Walter Camp's Daily Dozen, which was then so popular. And breathing exercises had the very special merit that they could be used in bed while I was waiting for sleep.

Experimenting with this idea, I began breathing on successive nights in as many different ways as I could think of. *Somewhat to my surprise I found that almost any variation of my normal unconscious breathing, if continued for some time, would bring on feelings of fatigue and drowsiness, though I noticed that certain types of breathing brought drowsiness much more quickly than others. So gradually I concentrated on the two or three most effective types.*

Imaginary Fireworks

In addition to using fatigue, one other idea for wooing sleep occurred to me, and I determined to try it, even though it did seem rather silly and not very promising. I had read that primitive peoples believed that their spirits actually left their bodies during sleep, thus accounting for the remarkable experiences of their dreams. So as I lay in bed I would imagine that I could see my spirit rising from my body and floating away. This did not interfere with my breathing exercises, and my tests left no doubt that it did actually aid in bringing sleep.

But the idea of my spirit floating away seemed so foolish that I decided to see whether something else would be just as effective. As a somewhat similar device, I tried watching imaginary fireworks, seeing the big rockets shooting up and bursting and the fireballs floating lazily down. This proved to be just as good for sleep-production, so I adopted imaginary fireworks as part of my nightly sleep-wooing procedure.

Using the best types of breathing control which I had discovered in combination with the imaginary fireworks proved to be all that I needed to assure me of sleep. I dropped the use of the sleeping powders entirely, and in a short time completely regained my normal health. But the very success of my experiments had aroused my curiosity and posed a number of questions which I was not satisfied to leave unanswered.

Some of these questions I found were not easy to answer. If the only effect of controlled breathing was to produce fatigue, then why should some types prove so much more effective than others in bringing sleep? And in any case, why should the slight fatigue produced by altered breathing be such an effective sleep producer? And what was there about watching imaginary fireworks that made it unquestionably helpful in bringing sleep, while the counting of imaginary sheep which I had often tried gave little if any help? After all, was there any sound reason why either the fireworks or the sheep should help to bring sleep, or was it only imagination?

How It Worked for Others

There was one question to which I got a very prompt answer. I wondered whether my procedures would work equally well when used by some other person. So I asked two of my sons, one at that time just beginning his medical studies and the other a business man, to try out my method of bringing sleep by watching imaginary fireworks while using certain types of controlled breathing. From both the report came back, "It works."

So it appeared that I had discovered a new and usable method of bringing sleep which had released me from an apparently hopeless quandary. If this were true, then were there not in all probability many other people in need of similar release?

Here the question arose, was my method indeed new? Certainly it seemed likely that someone would have hit upon the same or similar procedures, possibly long ago. To answer this question I read all of the popular books on sleep. They offered much advice on beds, bedrooms, ventilation, bedtime snacks, and other incidental matters. Some offered a collection of tricks gathered from various sources, leaving the reader to select those he fancied. Among these more or less magic tricks it was interesting to note the occasional occurrence of a variation of breathing or a peculiar use of the eyes. Usually, however, the author of the book did not regard these as aids to sleep, and often he did not appear to be aware of their presence. As for a systematic consideration of the psychological and physiological factors involved in the approach of sleep, these books did not even suggest it.

Several of the sleep books placed great emphasis on the need of learning to relax as a means of bringing sleep, usually basing this emphasis on the fact that relaxation reduces the nerve impulses coming to the brain from the muscles. Yet I had been

B

completely successful in putting myself to sleep before I read these books, and I had not given any thought at all to relaxation. Instead of answering my previous questions these books had only brought up an additional question. Why had the authors of these books considered efforts to relax so necessary, while I had so easily put myself to sleep without a thought of relaxation?

The Role of Carbon Dioxide

Looking further afield for answers to my questions I bought several books on physiology by such authors as W. B. Cannon, Best and Taylor, and Carlson and Johnson. From these I began to get some light on my questions. Most important, I learned of the part played by carbon dioxide in the chemistry of the body, and how its action is related to breathing. I realized that my controlled breathing was of a pattern which could only result in reduced ventilation with an increased retention of carbon dioxide which is associated with the relaxation unconsciously preceding normal sleep, the relaxation which various writers on sleep had sought to produce by conscious effort. I had always regarded carbon dioxide as merely one of the body's waste products. Now I discovered that modern physiologists give it a rank equal to the wonder-working hormones and other essential body chemicals. Indeed, the body's survival for even ten minutes depends on the precision by which the carbon dioxide circulating within the blood is controlled.

The first adequate discussion of sleep which I came upon in my reading was in "Fundamentals of Physiology," by Dr. Elbert Tokay. This book was especially helpful because it directed me to the work of Dr. Nathaniel Kleitman of the University of Chicago. Dr. Kleitman's book, "Sleep and Wakefulness," opened the whole field of sleep problems and sleep knowledge. Much subsequent searching has failed to find another book which can approach it as a complete and scientific treatment of sleep. But Dr. Kleitman evidently did not make it a primary purpose of his study to discover what natural resources the body and mind have within themselves for voluntarily inducing sleep, and his book, though practically an encyclopedia of sleep, would probably not help the average reader very much in meeting the problem of wakefulness.

Dr. Kleitman's bibliography of fourteen hundred references indicated the great number of books and articles published on sleep and related subjects, and the vast amount of material which I had yet to explore in my search. It was in fact only toward the end of a two-thousand-mile trip, searching well-known libraries for material on sleep, that I turned up the first lead on one of my questions. A book in the library of Wittenberg College published many years ago suggested a reason why watching imaginary fireworks should be more effective in bringing sleep than counting imaginary sheep. The difference turned out to be, when finally traced down, probably a reflex effect from the position of the eyes.

I found only one report of an attempt to evaluate scientifically the various means of bringing sleep without the use of drugs. This was an unpublished thesis in the library of Ohio State University. Unfortunately in this study no attention was given to the body's own resources, and the devices selected for testing were not such as could be made available to a person in his own bedroom.

For several years past my time has been largely spent in searching professional journals in the fields of physiology and medicine for material having a bearing on sleep. In these journals are to be found reports of many recent investigations which have not yet been published in book form. A number of these investigations, though in most cases they were made in the study of other problems, have developed facts of great significance in connection with the production of sleep. References to these reports will be found in various parts of this book. They have supplied answers to many questions, and also furnished striking scientific support for the sleep-producing procedures which had been developed in my experiments.

Summary: Four Simple Aids to Help You Sleep

The purpose of these procedures, briefly stated, is to utilize four aids: (1) through controlled breathing, the nerve-quieting and relaxing effects of carbon dioxide, (2) the drowsiness-producing effect of eye position, (3) preoccupation of the mind by mental picture-forming, and as a bonus by-product of these, (4) the basic sleep-producing condition, fatigue.

Why have these natural sleep-producing factors not previously been used in effective combination?

Apparently it has not occurred to anyone to ascertain what natural resources the body and mind have within themselves for inducing sleep by conscious effort. The easy procedures by which these natural resources can be called into action are described in the following chapters, and full instructions are given for putting them into successful use for bringing sleep.

3. A new use of breathing to aid sleep

Maximum inhalation	5 pints	"Complementary air" For large increases
Ordinary breathing	1 pint	"Tidal air" Quiet breathing
Maximum exhalation	2 pints	"Reserve air" For moderate increases
Air which can not be exhaled from the lungs	2 pints	"Residual air" Always retained

Figure 1. Lung capacity

The Air In Our Lungs

Our lungs provide us with an enormous reserve capacity for breathing, both in the volume of air taken in at each breath and also in the number of breaths a minute. Many people live in good health and breathe without inconvenience after one lung has been completely removed, the other lung fully meeting their need for oxygen under ordinary conditions. They feel their handicap only in severe exertion.

The total air capacity of the lungs of the average person is approximately ten pints. Of this total only one pint is breathed in and out in ordinary quiet breathing. Two pints of air remain in the lungs at all times and cannot be breathed out, even when an effort is made to empty the lungs. During quiet breathing an additional two pints is retained. Thus the lungs ordinarily keep a reserve of four pints of air to ensure a continuing supply of oxygen to the blood. Including this reserve, the lungs in quiet breathing are filled to only half their full capacity. The other half, an additional five pints, is used only when a larger supply of oxygen is needed by the body, as in vigorous exercise, though by voluntary control this extra capacity can be used at any time.

When compared with the total capacity of the lungs, taking breaths of only one pint seems to be very limited breathing. But this amount, taken sixteen or eighteen times a minute, fully meets the requirements of the body when it is at rest. In fact, even at this rate, air when breathed gives up only about one-fifth of its total content of oxygen. This amount is sufficient to fully charge the blood's oxygen carriers, the red corpuscles. Consequently breathing a larger amount of air would not increase the amount of oxygen carried by the blood or the amount used by the body.

How You Use Carbon Dioxide

The oxygen brought into our bodies by breathing is combined with certain elements in our food to produce heat and energy. This combination of oxygen with food elements is actually a form of burning, even thought it is accomplished in the body without the high heat of fire. Usually we describe this chemical process by saying that the food elements are oxidized. Our foods are composed principally of carbon and hydrogen. When the carbon in foods combines with oxygen it forms carbon dioxide. This is written by the chemist as CO_2, one atom of carbon combined with two atoms of oxygen. When the hydrogen in foods combines with oxygen it forms water, which the chemist writes as H_2O, two atoms of hydrogen, one of oxygen. This water is used by the body to supplement the liquids which are taken as drinks. The carbon dioxide, being a gas, mixes freely with the air in the lungs, and most of it is carried away in the breath.

While our incoming breaths are bringing in our needed supply of oxygen, our outgoing breaths are performing another essential service by carrying away the surplus of carbon dioxide which is produced in the body. These two functions of breathing will both be discussed in fuller detail in following sections of this book.

Until quite recently carbon dioxide was commonly regarded as purely a waste product, something to be gotten rid of as promptly as possible. As more recent studies have brought better knowledge of the marvelously complex chemical processes that are carried on in the body it has been found that while an excess of carbon dioxide is produced and breathed out through the lungs, large quantities of it are retained in the body and used in many important ways. Physicians now recognize that even minor variations in the carbon dioxide content of the blood may be highly significant.

One use the body makes of carbon dioxide is in maintaining the balance between acid and alkali. Carbon dioxide combines readily with water to form carbonic acid, a mild acid not to be confused with carbolic acid. Since an excess of carbon dioxide is constantly being produced, it is always available when needed to counteract excess alkali. Also, with equal facility it can be quickly thrown out of the body in the breath, thus reducing excess acidity. A proper acid-alkali balance is extremely important in the body, is in fact necessary to life. And carbon dioxide plays a most important part in the maintenance of this balance.

A second use of carbon dioxide in the body is in the regulation of breathing. We would naturally suppose that our unconscious breathing increases or decreases in response to the need of oxygen in the body. But this is true only under unusual conditions, such as severe exertion. Under ordinary conditions when the blood returns to the lungs after circulating through the body it still contains a large part of the oxygen with which it started out. The different organs of the body have simply used what they needed from the large excess supply which the blood was carrying. Under these conditions a little more or less oxygen in the blood makes hardly any difference in the body. In fact the oxygen in the blood has to be reduced by more than two-thirds before its lack can be felt. But any change in the carbon dioxide content of the blood changes the acid-alkali balance. In order to maintain this balance closely the respiratory center of the brain is highly sensitive to changes in the blood's carbon dioxide content, and it quickly increases or decreases involuntary breathing in order to remove more, or to retain more, of the carbon dioxide. Because the respiratory center responds so quickly to a change in the carbon dioxide content of the blood, carbon dioxide gives a much more exact control of unconscious breathing than oxygen could give. In tests it has been found that an increase of as little as one-fifth of one per cent of carbon dioxide in the arterial blood will cause a full doubling of the amount of air breathed per minute.

The question now arises, if breathing control is automatic and is regulated by the amount of carbon dioxide in the blood, how is it possible for us voluntarily to control our breathing in order to bring sleep?

The answer is that breathing forms an outstanding exception among the automatic processes of the body, being subject to double control. Conscious control can be substituted for unconscious control whenever we wish. The beating of our hearts is not subject to such double control. The movements of our stomachs and the secretion of the gastric juices, like the processes that maintain the body temperature, are entirely beyond voluntary control. We are not even aware of them. Yet breathing, which is equally essential to life, can be to a large extent purposely controlled. It can be greatly increased or diminished, or even stopped entirely for short periods.

Breath Control by Speakers, Singers

Why did nature make such an exception in the case of breathing? Or, how did it happen that in the course of evolution such a double control was developed? No doubt it was through attempts to use the breath for the purpose of producing sounds, a use which has now been very highly developed. It is evident at once that speaking would be impossible if breathing continued steadily, like the heart beats. Public speakers and singers develop breath control to a high degree. Athletes find it very important, especially swimmers and divers. So we see that conscious or voluntary control of breathing is not anything new or strange. It is a part of our daily living, so much so that we have come to take it as a matter of course and are no longer aware of it. Though we use it purposely but unconsciously, as we do many of our body faculties, there is no reason why we should not with conscious purpose continue to develop it and learn to adapt it for still other helpful uses. One possible use, to produce sleep, is the central concern of this book.

Experiments with voluntary alterations of breathing have shown that certain types of controlled breathing are highly effective in bringing sleep. In the following chapters these special types of breathing will be described in detail, so that it will be easy to learn them.

Diagrams of three types are shown to give clear mental pictures of the distinguishing features of each type, and of its operation in use. These diagrams should be studied carefully in connection with Figure 1. As a preparation for the use of each type in bringing sleep, it should be practiced in advance until it can be followed easily, almost automatically.

Summary: You Can Start It All in Bed

The proper place to practice these breathing exercises is in bed, where the body can be completely at ease. For greater freedom of breathing it is better to lie on the side, either right or left, as preferred. A pillow should be used which is just high enough to keep the neck straight. The head should be thrown slightly back, rather than forward. This affords freer breathing and helps to relax the muscles of the throat and of the eyes. Closing the eyes will help to center attention on the breathing.

All muscles of the body should be voluntarily relaxed as com-pletely as possible. Raising an arm or a leg and letting it drop limply may help in finding a relaxed position. If the body is in a state of habitual muscular tension, voluntary relaxation may be difficult, or incomplete. It is advised here only as a starter. More complete relaxation will come unconsciously as the breathing exercises are carried out, because, as explained in chapter 11, the carbon dioxide accumulated by reduced breathing exerts a strong relaxing influence as it is carried by the blood to all parts of the body.

A comfortable bed, a darkened room, absence of noise, freedom from disturbance, all these must be given attention, for they are very important aids to sleep. While it is important to avoid these external disturbances, the most serious interference with sleep usually comes from conditions that exist in the body and in the mind. Our first attention will be given to these conditions, which can be controlled effectively by the breathing exercises with their auxiliary features as outlined in the following chapters.

4. Let's start breathing
our way to sleep

Designation	Quantity	Breathing at rest	Three maximum breaths 15—20 seconds	Breath-holding 40 seconds, more or less
Complementary air	5 pints	(Not used in controlled breathing)		
Tidal air	1 pint			
Reserve air	2 pints			
Residual air	2 pints			

Figure 2. First Type of Breathing

(1) Maximum Breaths, (2) Breath-Holding

It is best to begin voluntary control of breathing by using periods of maximum breaths alternating with periods of breath-holding. Lying on your side in bed, inhale until the abdomen is fully expanded and the chest lifted as far as possible, then exhale completely, being sure to draw in the abdomen strongly at the end of the exhalation in order to expel as much air as possible from the lungs. The abdomen should then be allowed to relax completely, but without inhaling.

After an instant in this relaxed condition, with the lungs as empty as possible, start to inhale again in the same way, and

43

repeat the exhalation and relaxing, until you have done this three times.

At the end of the first period of three maximum breaths, when the lungs are as empty as possible and the abdomen fully relaxed, a period of breath-holding is begun. In this condition the breath is held, neither inhaling nor exhaling, until discomfort arises and the impulse to breathe again can no longer be easily resisted.

When this point of discomfort is reached a second period of maximum breaths is begun, consisting of three maximum inhalations, each exhaled completely, as described above. These three maximum breaths are followed by a second period of breath-holding, to be continued as long as possible without discomfort. Several periods of breath-holding, alternated with groups of three maximum breaths, will be necessary.

The Object: To Retain More of the Body's Carbon Dioxide While Still Supplying Ample Oxygen

Tests under carefully controlled conditions have shown that while oxygen continues to be absorbed from the lungs during breath-holding, very little of the carbon dioxide produced from this oxygen is returned to the lungs, most of it remaining in the blood and body tissues.

No more than three consecutive maximum breaths in each period are recommended. The three deep breaths largely restore the oxygen content of the blood and remove enough carbon dioxide to reduce somewhat the impulse toward continuous breathing. This makes it possible to hold the breath longer and so gain an increased accumulation of carbon dioxide in the blood and throughout the body.[1]

---

[1] The carbon dioxide reduces alkalinity and slows the activity of the nerves and the brain, readying them for the onset of sleep. If continued to more than three breaths, deep breathing would greatly reduce the carbon dioxide content of the blood, and correspondingly increase its alkalinity. This increase of alkalinity would heighten the activity of the nerves and also of the brain, making them much more sensitive to excitement or stimulation of any kind. With only three maximum breaths together this increase of sensitivity is not great enough to excite the nerves or disturb mental quiet.

No Need for Fear

While holding the breath, that is, refraining from breathing when the lungs have expelled their air, the lungs should be kept as empty as possible, so that the air in them will absorb only a small amount of carbon dioxide from the blood. No fear need be felt that the body will suffer from lack of oxygen during these breath-holding periods. At the start of breath-holding the blood contains four or five times as much oxygen as the body will use during the breath-holding period of forty seconds, and residual air which cannot be expelled from the lungs contains a considerable additional amount. The three maximum breaths which follow restore approximately the same condition for the start of the next period of breath-holding.

Successful control of the breathing as described can be secured most easily if some means is used to divert the mind from the breathing. Allusion was made in Chapter 2 to the device of watching imaginary fireworks, and use could be made of various other devices, but after extensive testing nothing better has been found for general use than the mental repetition of the following Mother Goose lines. They should be memorized, so that they almost seem to repeat themselves. With this repetition to occupy the mind the breath can be held longer and the accumulation of carbon dioxide in the body carried that much further.

> Rock-a-bye, baby, up in the tree top.
> When the wind blows, baby's cradle will rock;
> Baby's cradle will rock, baby's cradle will rock.
> With the tree's drowsy swing baby's cradle will rock.
>
> Since the big bough is not likely to break,
> Fear of a fall won't keep baby awake;
> Won't keep baby awake, won't keep baby awake.
> No disquieting care will keep baby awake.

Let Your Mind Form Pictures

Tests have shown that diversion of the mind is most complete when it is engaged in forming a series of definite and varied mental pictures. This is explained more fully in Appendix A. While repeating the lines above, therefore, clear mental pictures should be formed of the tree, the baby, the cradle, the rocking motion, the sturdy bough, the tree's swing in the wind. The tree should be imagined as a tall one, standing almost overhead. This will cause the eyes to turn upward, just as if looking up into an actual tree, in this way affording an additional aid to sleep. In all the breathing exercises the eyes should be turned upward. In the periods of maximum breaths this can be made easy by repeating the words "eyes up" with each breath, the word *eyes* while inhaling, and *up* while exhaling.

The Mother Goose lines above have been chosen partly because they are already associated in everyone's mind with sleep. They have been freely altered to keep the eyes directed upward and to give additional suggestion of sleep. They have also been extended to make two four-line stanzas, so that their repetition will occupy a full period of breath-holding. For greater peace of mind the baby's tragic fall has been sidestepped. These lines have a rhythm which matches well with the beating of the heart, and in their mental repetition each accented syllable can be made to correspond with a beat of the heart. This will give uniformity to the speed of repetition and serve as a measure of the length of time that the breath is held. The heart beats can be easily followed by placing the finger tips on the pulse at the wrist.

No unpleasant effort should be made to continue a period of breath-holding until the two stanzas can be completed. When the desire to breathe again becomes urgent, the mental repetition and the breath-holding should be broken off and another period of three maximum breaths started. If occasionally it is found comfortable to hold the breath somewhat longer, the last two lines or all of the second stanza, can be repeated a second time.

When going to sleep immediately after eating, the breath-holding time is apt to be noticeably shortened. When this occurs it is better to take four maximum breaths in each period instead of three. This extra breath supplies the extra oxygen used in digesting and assimilating food.

The two stanzas given are to be used over and over, each period of breath-holding being started with the first line of the first stanza. This monotony of repeating the same words is in itself a minor aid in bringing sleep, and our aim is to utilize everything that will help us go to sleep.

The periods of breath-holding will, of course, build up a strong desire to breathe again, but this will be relieved by the three following maximum breaths. While these three breaths almost completely restore the oxygen supply of the blood, they only partly remove the carbon dioxide accumulated in the body tissues during a period of breath-holding. Consequently the end result of a series of these alternating periods of maximum breaths and breath-holding is to accumulate more carbon dioxide in the tissues of the body than they would ordinarily contain, causing drowsiness and relaxation. The physiological effects of breath-holding and of the increase of carbon dioxide which it brings in the body are discussed more fully in chapter 16, and in Appendix B.

How Fatigue Can Help

A second very important effect of the alternate maximum breaths and breath-holding is the production of fatigue, which is a basic aid in bringing sleep. Physiologists agree that it is not necessary to exercise all the muscles of the body to produce a feeling of fatigue. Use of only one group of muscles can make the whole body feel tired. Doctors often use maximum breathing as an aid in diagnosis, and they have found that it will produce fatigue very quickly. The periods of breath-holding also add to the feeling of fatigue because effort is required to restrain the impulse to breathe.

The maximum breaths and breath-holding should be continued through four to eight periods of maximum breaths and three to seven periods of breath-holding, always beginning and ending with a period of three maximum breaths.

After a few periods of maximum breaths and breath-holding it will be noticed that the three maximum breaths do not quite relieve the desire to breathe which is built up by the breath-holding, so that there is an inclination to inhale a fourth time, and a slight effort is required to start the succeeding period of breath-holding. It is at this point, and for the purpose of avoiding this increased effort, that a change is made to the second type of breathing. This change should not be made, however, until after a considerable period of practice with the first type of breathing. When the first type of breathing has become practically automatic, the second type can be taken up at the point where the first type begins to require increased effort.

The first type of breathing, because it does require some effort, helps to divert the mind from its previous lines of thought, which, if they are allowed to intrude, will hinder the approach of sleep. But this effort, if continued too long, may defeat its own purpose, that of bringing sleep. Consequently, while learning this type of breathing, the beginner should continue it only to the point of definite fatigue, and then rest for a few minutes before taking it up again. This period of rest often passes unexpectedly into sleep.

Summary: If At First You Don't Succeed—

Except in stubborn cases, repetition of the first type of breathing, with the accumulating fatigue and other effects of the procedure as outlined, will usually be sufficient to bring sleep. It can be continued to any length without harm or discomfort, and whether it brings sleep or not, it should be faithfully practiced on several successive nights until it can be carried out almost automatically. Only when this training period is completed should the second type of breathing be attempted. But after both types have been learned, using the two in combination will assure quicker and more certain results.

5. Reduce your tension
by this simple method

Designation	Quantity	Previous breath-holding	Three maximum breaths 15—20 seconds	Minimum breathing Indefinite time
Complementary air	5 pints	Not used in second type of breathing		
Tidal air	1 pint			
Reserve air	2 pints			
Residual air	2 pints			

Figure 3. Second Type of Breathing

(1) Maximum Breaths, (2) Minimum Breathing

This second type of breathing is begun by following the last period of three maximum breaths in the first type with a period of minimum breathing, this minimum breathing taking the place of the breath-holding used in the first type of breathing. Minimum breathing means breathing in and out so slightly that the movement of the air in the nostrils is just perceptible. This minimum breathing must be very shallow and the breaths very short. A good way to time the breaths is by placing the fingers on the pulse and breathing in on one beat and out on the next. Care must be used to avoid filling the lungs. They should be almost as empty as during the periods of breath-holding, and the abdomen should be fully relaxed. These short, shallow breaths are to be continued until a strong urge to breathe more deeply is felt. Then another period of maximum breaths is started, consisting of three very full breaths, each exhaled completely, as in the first type of breathing. Another period of minimum breathing follows the maximum breaths, and is continued as long as it is comfortable.

Object: To Increase Carbon Dioxide Without Producing Nervous Tension

The air taken in with each short breath should be just about enough to fill the air passages from the nose to the air sacs of the lungs. These passages are called by physiologists the dead spaces, because the air in them does not reach the respiratory part of the lungs to supply oxygen and carry away carbon dioxide. This dead space is equal to about one-third of an ordinary quiet breath. So when the breaths are only one-third as deep as in ordinary quiet breathing the effect is almost the same as if the breath were held completely. However, these shallow breaths give relief to the breathing muscles, because minimum breathing requires less effort than holding the breath for an equal length of time. This permits an increased accumulation of carbon dioxide in the body without disturbing the composure and relaxation needed for sleep.

A Poem to Match the Breaths

In this second type of breathing a long-familiar poem is repeated mentally as an aid in keeping the breaths short and shallow during the periods of minimum breathing. This repetition helps, too, to keep the thoughts from wandering to disturbing subjects, and it furnishes mental pictures which turn the eyes upward, two aids which are important in all the breathing exercises. Here again liberties have been taken with the usual version of the poem by substituting a third stanza better suited to our purposes. This poem carries strong suggestions of night and bedtime. It is "Twinkle, twinkle, little star," and recalls pleasant memories to almost everyone. It was written to express the thoughts of a little child as he looked at a star, and this idea should be carried out in the mental repetition of the lines, the eyes being directed upward to an imaginary star. The lines as given below should be memorized.

The meter of these lines is such that they fit well with the short, shallow breaths. Each accented syllable is followed by one unaccented syllable, except at the end of each line, where an accented syllable stands alone. In the repetition the first accented syllable goes with an inhalation, the second accented syllable with an exhalation, and so on. In this way each line begins with an inhalation and ends with an exhalation. For the beginner it is well to time the repetition with the pulse as suggested above, one beat going with an inhalation and the next with an exhalation.

> Twinkle, twinkle, little star,
> How I wonder what you are,
> Up above the world so high,
> Like a diamond in the sky.
>
> When the blazing sun has set,
> And the grass with dew is wet,
> Then you show your little light,
> Twinkle, twinkle, all the night.
>
> Gleaming brightly overhead,
> While I'm warm and snug in bed,
> You will through my window peep,
> Twinkling still while I'm asleep.

If the short breaths are kept sufficiently shallow while repeating these three stanzas, they will build up a strong desire to take a fuller breath. To relieve this desire a group of three maximum breaths should be taken in the usual manner, to be followed by a period of short breaths as before.

Striking proof that the repetition of familiar lines is an effective means of quieting the mind has come from the recent discovery of a new type of brain waves. These are the kappa waves, often called thought waves, because they are believed to be associated with the thought activities of the brain. They have been found to be at their lowest point during the repetition of perfectly familiar material.

You Are Now Halfway to Sleep

A common sign that sleep is approaching is the intrusion of transient, irrelevant mental pictures along with or in place of the purposeful picture of the twinkling star which is being consciously held in the mind's eye. These uninvited mental pictures which intrude in this way are characteristic of an intermediate mental state halfway between sleep and wakefulness. As a rule, when they appear, continuing the breathing procedure a little while longer will bring sleep.

Another signal that sleep is near is a momentary forgetfulness of the perfectly familiar lines that are being mentally repeated. This is simply a brief stopping of the normal activity of the mind. Presumably it is very similar to what happens when one actually passes into sleep. If it continued a little longer it would no doubt be sleep, or at least it would become sleep. After such an interruption prompt resumption of the repetition and minimum breathing will usually bring sleep promptly.

Itching sensations about the nose and mouth sometimes occur when sleep is approaching. The cause of these sensations is not understood, but it is believed that they have a definite connection with the coming of sleep. Consequently the wise thing to do is not to take them as interruptions or disturbances, but to regard them as reassuring indications that sleep is on the way.

Under favorable conditions this second type of breathing, when carried through with the additional aids recommended, will in most cases bring sleep. If occasionally it fails, there is an additional type of breathing which can be used to supplement the first two types and to add to their effectiveness. It has been especially devised to give stronger control of disturbing thoughts. When persistent wakefulness is clearly due to a state of high mental tension, this supplemental type of breathing will be found highly effective. Through the use of a carefully devised system of mental picture forming it affords an unequalled degree of thought control. (The supplemental type of breathing is omitted from the main text of the book and printed in the appendix, because it will not often be needed and because its explanation is necessarily somewhat lengthy and its mastery requires memorizing the numbers used. However, it will not be found difficult to master, and at a convenient time it should be learned and held in reserve ready for use if needed.) The supplemental type of breathing is not intended for beginners and should not be undertaken until the other types of breathing have been used over a considerable period and have become perfectly familiar, almost automatic.

You Should Rest When Tired

During the sleep-training period, whenever definite fatigue is felt, a short interval of rest should be taken. During this rest interval the breathing should be forgotten and left to unconscious, automatic control. The thoughts should be turned to pleasant and undisturbing subjects. When the breathing muscles are rested, or if the mind persistently turns to thoughts that are disturbing, controlled breathing should be started again, beginning with the first type and proceeding through the second type as before. But do not be surprised if you wake later and find that sleep came unawares during the rest period. Frequently, when the breathing exercises have prepared both the body and the mind, merely stopping all conscious effort will bring sleep.

While these breathing procedures afford a very effective means of bringing sleep, they are by no means a knock-out method, and their effects are entirely different from those of the brain-stupefying drugs in sleeping pills. These drugs disrupt the chemical processes of the brain to the point where it is no longer able to maintain consciousness, so that a sleep-like stupor intervenes in spite of efforts that may be made to stay awake. By contrast the method here outlined brings sleep through a combination of certain mild and perfectly natural and wholesome influences that can be brought to bear on the brain, with no risk of the long-continued and sometimes permanent dulling of the mind which may result from sleeping pills.

This milder method has two great advantages. The first advantage is that it brings real sleep, with all its natural restorative value for both mind and body, which the stupor of sleeping pills can never equal. This follows from the fact that the procedures used merely initiate sleep, all the different sleep-inducing factors losing their effect the instant that consciousness is lost in sleep, so that the natural recuperation of sleep proceeds unhindered by any depressing influence. The second advantage of this milder method is that there is no danger that this method of inducing sleep will ever be used as a pain-killer or a deadener of the senses to substitute for the proper treatment of disease. It is ineffective for this purpose, and so allows wakefulness to continue as a warning that medical treatment is needed to remove the cause of the pain.

Summary: Remember, the Effect Is Cumulative. Combine, Repeat!

The principle of using a combination of influences in order to produce a cumulative effect has long been recognized in doctors' prescriptions, which often contain several different drugs that act together to produce an effect greater than the sum of their effects would be if they were given separately.

So in carrying out these instructions it must be remembered that the purpose is to apply a combination of mild sleep-producing influences, and that it is only in combination that their full effects can be realized. The neglect of any single factor may defeat the purpose of the combination.

The relaxing of the muscles and the quieting of the nerves by the carbon dioxide retained in the body; the fatigue produced by

the control of breathing; the reflex effect of turning the eyes upward; the effective diversion and preoccupation of the mind by
the repetitions and the forming of mental pictures; even the mild
autosuggestions of sleep and of the sheltered security of childhood
which are called up by the simple rhymes given for repetition; all
these are useful elements in the combination designed to bring
sleep.

6. Yet another way to
bring on sleep easily

(1) Many Maximum Breaths, (2) Minimum Breaths

For some people, and under some conditions, it may be found simpler and easier to bring sleep by starting the breathing exercises, not with three maximum breaths, but with several times that number, a dozen, two dozen, or more, not forgetting to repeat mentally with each maximum breath the words "eyes up" and to hold the eyes steadily upward, and not stopping until a very definite effort is required for continuing the maximum inhalations. This repetition and the effort of maintaining the maximum breaths will at the same time serve to keep the mind fully occupied. At the end of this long series of maximum breaths, instead of a period of breath-holding, as in the first type of breathing, it is better to use a period of minimum breaths, as in the second type of breathing, accompanying this minimum breathing with mental repetition of the same stanzas used there.

The basis in brain physiology for the long period of maximum breathing used in this optional type of procedure may be stated as follows: Scientific experiments have demonstrated that it is of great importance to the normal activity of the brain that the carbon dioxide content of its blood supply should not vary too much. Maximum breathing throws off an increased amount of carbon dioxide from the blood as it passes through the lungs, so that the blood then returns to the brain with much less than its normal content of carbon dioxide. However, as part of what the late Dr. W. B. Cannon called "the wisdom of the body," the brain has its own automatic protection against excessive reduction in its supply of carbon dioxide.

Your Brain Is Always on Guard

The brain itself is constantly producing carbon dioxide. In fact, it produces much more in proportion to its weight than any other part of the body. Ordinarily this carbon dioxide is carried away in the circulating blood as rapidly as it is formed. But when the blood coming to the brain begins to fall below its normal content of carbon dioxide, the brain's small blood vessels immediately contract, slowing up the flow of blood, and in this way accumulating enough of its own production of carbon dioxide to maintain the normal content.

While the brain's circulation is slowed to increase its carbon dioxide the brain still continues to use oxygen from the slowly flowing blood as rapidly as if the blood were flowing at its usual rate. The effect of this is to cause the blood, which ordinarily carries a large surplus of oxygen through the brain, to become relatively poor in oxygen. When this reduction of oxygen content reaches a certain point the brain can no longer obtain its normal oxygen supply and is obliged to slow down its activities.

At this point, with the brain's activity slowed by the low oxygen from restricted blood circulation, if we suddenly reduce breathing to a minimum, this stops the rapid throwing off of carbon dioxide by the lungs, and sends blood to the brain with much more than even its normal supply of carbon dioxide. The brain's own output of carbon dioxide is then added to this, so that for a little time, until its blood vessels can dilate and increase the blood flow, the brain is subject not only to a low oxygen content in its circulating blood but also to a doubly increased amount of carbon dioxide, adding a second strong influence to slow the brain's activity. Under favorable conditions this combination of low oxygen and high carbon dioxide can reduce the brain's activity almost to the sleep level. With a continuation of the minimum breathing to maintain the high content of carbon dioxide in the blood, in cases where there was only a moderate tendency to wakefulness, sleep may come almost immediately.

Why You Twitch

Here the question naturally arises, if this is an easier way to bring sleep, why was it not made the standard procedure. The first answer is that the standard procedure was planned, not primarily for speed or convenience, but to afford the greatest possible effectiveness in cases of stubborn or persistent wakefulness. Where there is likely to be difficulty in getting to sleep it is usually best to stick to the standard procedure. A second answer is that many people cannot use this optional procedure because their brains are not adequately protected against the effects of prolonged maximum breathing. In some cases this may be only a temporary condition, but in others it is a permanent inborn characteristic. For people who have this limitation, prolonging the maximum breathing is liable to start involuntary muscular twitches which will effectively drive sleep away.

These muscular twitches are caused by the increased alkalinity of the blood circulating in the brain. In health the blood is always slightly alkaline, and the degree of this alkalinity is regulated largely by the amount of carbon dioxide which the blood is carrying. Over-breathing reduces the carbon dioxide and increases the alkalinity. At a certain degree of increased alkalinity the nerve centers of the brain become so excitable that they begin to send out contraction impulses to the muscles without waiting for orders from the conscious part of the mind. When for any reason the small blood vessels of the brain do not contract promptly in response to over-breathing, they fail to slow the blood flow and consequently fail to maintain the normal proportion of carbon dioxide. With the carbon dioxide content of the blood lowered and its alkalinity correspondingly increased, the nerve centers of the brain necessarily become highly excitable. So when a person's brain does not have adequate automatic regulation of blood flow he cannot use long periods of maximum breathing to bring sleep.

There is a very simple method of reducing breathing which is sometimes recommended as a means of bringing sleep. This method is simply to go to sleep while lying in a face-down position. In this position the weight of the body on the chest and the abdomen will hinder the movement of the breathing muscles and in this way reduce the amount of air breathed without requiring any voluntary effort. Where the difficult of going to sleep is slight, this method is often successful. However, it is not recommended, party because this face-down position is uncomfortable for most people, but more especially because the reduced breathing does not end with the coming of sleep but is carried on into the period of sleep, when breathing should be unobstructed. Persons who have been accustomed to go to sleep while lying face-down will be likely to find their sleep more restful if they will lie on the side and reduce their breathing by using the procedures earlier outlined. With these procedures, reduction of breathing is voluntary, and the reduction ceases as soon as sleep comes. Unconscious regulation then gives just the volume of breathing which is best for normal sleep.

In outlining the various procedures for bringing sleep, minor variations and adaptations have been suggested at several points. While the procedures given are believed likely to be most successful in the great majority of cases, there is no desire to rule out other possible procedures if they are so devised as to produce the desired physiological and psychological effects. These effects and the means to obtain them have been described in detail to give the user full and free command over their use, so that he may easily adapt them to his individual and temporary requirements. If the underlying principles are observed, the details of procedure may be varied.

Pick Your Own Lullaby—But Watch the Meter

As an illustration of possible adaptations, some may prefer to use other poems as substitutes for the rhymes which have been given for repetition. In making such changes two points should be kept in mind. First, the length of time required for repetition of the substitute should not vary greatly from the example given. Second, and more important, the same meter should be used. In the breath-holding periods this consists of one accented syllable alternating with two unaccented, (—uu—uu—) which when synchronized with the heartbeat regulates the speed of repetition and gauges the length of the breath-holding. In the periods of short breaths an accented syllable alternates with one unaccented, (—u—u—u—) which gives a quick movement and helps to keep the breaths short and the breathing shallow.

Various reasons might be found for preferring substitutes or revisions in place of the verses given. Those who think that the original ideas of "Twinkle, twinkle, little star" are now outmoded might prefer some such revision as follows:

> Twinkle, twinkle, little star,
> Now we know just what you are,
> Up above the world so high,
> Like an arc light in the sky.

> You are just another sun,
> Which through the heavens his course must run,
> But many billion miles away,
> You cannot change our night to day.

> Yet when our sun has sunk from sight
> We're glad to see your cheery light,
> And know you will your vigil keep
> All through the night while we're asleep.

7. How to control external disturbances

You Must Shut Off the Senses

In any plan to make sure of sleep, outside disturbances must be dealt with. These are disturbances that come through the senses, seeing and hearing being the most important.

Nature has provided a period of darkness in each twenty-four hours, during which most of our sleeping is done, and in which it is easy to avoid disturbances that come through the sense of sight. Fortunately, nature has provided us also with eyelids, so that even in the daytime we can stop seeing things by merely closing our eyes. But because bright light penetrates the eyelids to some extent, a sleeping room, if not dark, should at least have only subdued light. This can usually be secured by closing blinds, pulling down shades, or placing screens in front of open windows. Some stores sell "sleep shades" which can be worn to supplement the eyelids.

Unfortunately, nature has not provided us with earlids, and the organs of hearing have no natural means of effectively shielding themselves against the intrusion of sounds. It is true that we can become accustomed to certain types of sounds, so that they no longer disturb us seriously, but any unusual noise, whether louder or of a different kind, is likely to interfere with sleep. Even when noise does not keep one awake, it may make sleep lighter and less restful. Telephones and door bells within hearing are almost sure to keep one awake, if only by the knowledge that they are likely to ring. To make sure of sleep, bells within hearing must be muffled. Bells are often unattended while we go to market or to the movies. Is not one's sleep of equal importance?

Soundproofing of sleeping rooms with various kinds of insulation is well worth while. Doors are usually made of very thin wood and do not obstruct sound to any great extent. A sheet of insulating board fastened with a few tiny screws against a door leading into a hallway or into another room will greatly reduce noises from other parts of the house. Thin partitions can be similarly covered. A window next to the street may be covered in the same way during sleeping hours. Sound absorbing materials are now available that may be applied to walls and ceilings. A loose window sash or blind, being shaken irregularly by the wind, is often a cause of wakefulness. Proper fastenings, or even small wooden wedges, will stop the noise. If the sound of an electric fan or the ticking of an alarm clock is disturbing, heavy felt or sponge rubber under it will quiet it. Other occupants of the house who may be astir should be asked not to slam doors, speak in high-pitched tones, or walk with quick or heavy steps, but to keep the sleeper in mind.

Anyone For Home-made Ear Plugs?

After everything else has been done, an additional defense against noise can be obtained by soundproofing the ears. Various kinds of ear plugs have been devised. Some are on sale in drug stores and sleep shops. Sound-insulating ear muffs to be worn over the ears are available in some stores. In the absence of anything better, plugs of cotton or softened paraffin may be used. A durable and very effective ear plug can easily be made from a pencil-cap eraser. It should be of soft rubber and of a size to fit the ear. With a sharp knife or a razor blade, moistened, the solid part of the eraser is trimmed away until only the cup remains. Sharp corners are smoothed with a fine file or sandpaper. A dozen or so strands of wool crochet yarn are tied round with spool thread. With a thin sliver of wood or metal resting on this tie the strands of yarn are forced into the rubber cup. Scissors are used to trim the ends of the yarn flush with the rubber. There should be enough strands of yarn to fit moderately tight in the rubber cup, but not enough to bulge it. Holding the cup by the closed end, the open end is moistened slightly in the mouth and then forced firmly into the ear. A very small perforation in the bottom of the cup will ensure against uncomfortable air pressure in the ear. A pair of these plugs well fitted will materially dull the hearing and bring extra hours of sleep.

One Way to Drown Out Noises

Sometimes the best way to deal with intermittent noises is to drown them with a continuous noise. A person becomes accustomed to a moderate continuous noise, so that it is not disturbing, and other noises are not noticed. An electric fan can be used to produce a continuous noise, even when it is not needed for cooling. If its noise is not loud enough, it can be placed on a wood or metal support which will act as a sounding board. Removing felt or rubber pads under the fan base will make it still louder. To prevent the fan from "walking" off its support, cut surgeon's adhesive tape in lengths three times its width, fold these lengths into squares with the gum outward, and apply them under the fan's base. Placing the support of the fan in contact with the bedstead will make its noise seem still louder.

Too Hot or too Cold?

In addition to light and noise, uncomfortable heat or cold can be disturbing. Disturbance from cold is most likely to come from some part of the body not being warm enough, usually the feet. Bed socks, a hot-water bottle, or an electric heating pad should be available. For bald heads a nightcap will be helpful. Bedcovers must be adjusted according to the temperature of the bedroom, with preference given to covers of light weight. One should never go to bed in a warm room which will cool off during the night. Windows should be opened and the temperature reduced to a point at which it can be maintained through the night. Sixty degrees Fahrenheit is a good temperature for restful sleep. Where temperature cannot be controlled, and the room is likely to get cold during the night, an automatic electric blanket may be desirable.

If It's Too Hot to Sleep. Since many houses do not yet have hot weather air conditioning, sleep disturbance from heat may be difficult to deal with. Rooms on the first floor and those on the northeast corner of the house are likely to be coolest. Large shade trees on the south and west sides of a house and wide overhangs of the roof do much to reduce the heat, especially the accumulation of heat in the walls, which continues to be felt into the night. Proper ventilation of the attic is very important, and an attic fan is very effective for cooling the house during the night. Cooling a house at night and keeping the windows and doors closed during the day helps to keep the rooms from getting so hot during the day. The ideal solution of the heat problem is to insulate the bedroom and install a refrigerating type of air conditioner. It not only reduces the temperature but also dries the air, while its fan keeps the air in motion, so that it carries away the surplus heat of the body.

Too soft a mattress will greatly increase the discomfort of heat, though it is desirable to have the mattress soft enough not to press too firmly against the body at any one point. Two or three thicknesses of floor matting over the mattress, while yielding to pressure, will hold the mattress away from the body and afford coolness by permitting circulation of air. A pillow into which the head sinks can be made firmer and cooler by forcing the filler into one end and tucking the empty end under. An electric fan can be a great relief from heat, but it must not blow too directly on the body. Dispensing with pajamas and sleeping with only a sheet for cover, or with no cover at all, may be desirable on very hot nights. A canvas cot without mattress is the coolest of all beds, and a tent pitched in the back yard can be the coolest bedroom.

Another person sleeping in the same bed or in the same room may sometimes be a serious disturbance. A light sleeper may well have a bed, or better still, a room, all to himself.

Other Causes of Wakefulness

Perhaps one other outside source of disturbance should be mentioned. This is insects, particularly flies and mosquitoes. Where sleeping quarters are not screened this may be serious. And sometimes these insects get into screened quarters. Even one mosquito can spoil a night's sleep. Insect repellents and chemical sprays should be kept on hand to supplement screens. A hemisphere of mosquito netting framed with stiff wire and used as a head-and-shoulders canopy can be a valuable help. A great virtue of this appliance is that an insect inside it can be released by inverting it for a moment, with little disturbance to the would-be sleeper. The diameter of this canopy should be twenty-four to thirty inches, and several inches of netting should extend beyond the wire all round to make contact with the bed. If the wire framework is made of four half-circles with loops at the ends to hinge on rivets or bolts where they join, this canopy can be folded into small space.

Without debating whether foods and drinks are external or internal disturbances of sleep, their importance merits some attention. If there is a considerable interval between the last regular meal of the day and the time of retiring, and especially if there is considerable activity or intense application during this time, a moderate amount of food may be needed at bedtime to prevent the development of hunger during sleep. This food may be either liquid or solid, though it is to be noted that liquid in any considerable quantity taken at bedtime may disturb sleep by distention of the bladder. Sweets of any kind are apt to be slightly stimulating and so delay the onset of sleep. Cereals are better than sweets for a bedtime snack. A cup of hot milk seasoned with salt rather than sugar is a good bedtime drink. Its warmth gives a slight relaxing effect which aids sleep. *Except for this relaxation and the prevention of hunger, there is no food or drink known which possesses any peculiar effectiveness in producing sleep.*

Many soft drinks contain caffeine, the stimulating drug found

c

in coffee. Its effect is usually felt in one to two hours and may continue as long as eleven hours. Tea, cocoa, and chocolate contain similar stimulants. Anyone who is sensitive to these drugs should avoid taking them too near retiring. Alcohol does not affect all persons alike. For some it may be very disturbing to sleep if taken near bedtime, even in the diluted forms of beer and wine. The taking of thyroid extract may interfere with sleep, and for some persons even the use of certain types of nasal inhalers may be a hindrance.

In all these cases every individual is to a certain extent a law unto himself. He must determine, after trial, what is for him a hindrance to sleep, and what is a help.

8. How to benefit from the one-third of your life you spend in bed— how to pick your bed, mattress, and pillow

Where One-Third of Your Life Is Spent

How to Pick a Good Bed. Sleep can be made more certain and more refreshing by a good bed, and it can be made restless or impossible by a poor bed. What then are the characteristics of a good bed?

First of all, a bed must be neither too hard nor too soft. A hard bed concentrates the pressure of the body's weight on only a few points of the body, because the surface of a hard bed is usually in a flat plane which the body's surface, being curved, touches only at certain points. These points on the body are subject to sufficient pressure to impede the circulation of the blood, and in some cases to compress blood vessels and nerves. This will create discomfort or pain and cause disturbed sleep or wakefulness. Persons whose bones are well protected with flesh are least affected by a hard bed. Persons who sleep soundly often are able to get relief from the local pressure by changing their position without waking. Such persons often seem to rest better on a moderately firm bed. Persons whose bones are not so well protected, and persons who wake easily, are likely to rest better on a bed which is soft enough to yield easily to increased pressure, as this tends to equalize the pressure at all points of contact with the body.

A bed is too soft if it allows the body to sink down into it, forming a sort of mold that extends upward on all sides. This causes over-heating and lack of ventilation of the underside of the body, and makes relief by changing position much more difficult.

A clear distinction must be made between a soft bed and a sagging bed. A bed is soft when the top surface of the mattress yields to pressure without noticeably changing the bottom surface. A bed sags when pressure on the top surface of the mattress causes the bottom surface to yield almost as much as the top because of improper support under the mattress. A bony person or a person of slight weight may find a soft bed desirable, but a sagging bed is not suitable for anyone.

Once Upon a Mattress. Three methods are in common use for supporting mattresses. The most common is a series of coiled springs arranged side by side on a relatively firm support. These coils are connected at the top by links of wire so that they can yield individually to pressure from the mattress. The effect is to make a mattress seem softer and also to cause the mattress to adapt itself somewhat to the curves of the sleeper's body. A proper combination of thickness and softness of the mattress and strength and closeness of the coil springs will produce an excellent bed. If the springs are strong enough for proper support of the sleeper's weight they will not sag objectionably.

A second type of mattress support in common use is the woven-wire spring, sometimes a fabric of interconnected horizontal coils of fine wires stretched in a steel frame, and sometimes a series of connected wire links joined to the steel frame with short coil springs. In either type no one point can be depressed without pulling down all the surrounding surface. Such springs always produce a sagging bed. Stretching them tightly in the frame will reduce the sag but will not cure it.

A third type of mattress support is a solid board nearly the full size of the mattress. This is placed between the springs and the mattress, and its effect is to make the springs useless. Placed under coil springs the board is useless. Under woven springs the board may correct or reduce sag. Persons who prefer a hard, level bed should use such a board as the mattress support and discard the springs. Combined with the proper mattress, a board produces a good bed.

The inner-spring mattress now in such common use is simply a combination of two thin mattresses with coil springs between. What has been said about mattresses and coil springs applies also to this combination. When the mattresses are of sufficient thickness and of the right degree of firmness, and the coil springs are of the right strength and closely spaced, an inner-spring mattress can make an excellent bed. Such a mattress needs no additional springs. It should be placed on a full-size bed board or on stiff, closely spaced cross supports.

The author has slept for many years on a modified woven wire spring, and he believes it to be pretty near an ideal mattress support. It forms what might be called a contour bed, and allows the use of a firm mattress without causing uncomfortable pressure on the hips and shoulders. Two straps of heavy sheet metal are drawn tightly across under the wire network and fastened securely to the steel frame of the spring at each side. These straps are placed so that one gives support to the mattress just above the hips and the other just below the hips of the sleeper. This allows the mattress to yield under the hips and equalize the pressure which on a perfectly flat mattress is much greater at this point. The shoulders also are in a yielding area between the head of the bed and the upper of the two sheet metal straps. These straps do not prevent completely the tendency of the woven wire springs to sag, because they still permit the formation of a slight lengthwise trough in the center of the bed. But this can be easily overcome by placing a folded blanket or other padding over the center of the springs under the mattress. It should be added that this type of mattress support is better suited to single than to double beds.

With the body contour provided by these metal straps, there is no need for coil springs, either inside or outside the mattress. A cotton mattress about six inches thick will give ample softness if it is selected according to the weight of the sleeper. This combination of a body contour with an otherwise flat mattress is the aim of a new type of mattress which has a board in the center with inner springs above and below it, a cumbersome build-up which only approximates its purpose.

Bedcovers should always be chosen to give the desired warmth with the least possible weight. When sleeping in a cold room with several covers, the lightest should be placed next to the body and the heaviest outside. This makes it possible to adjust more exactly for the desired warmth. If the heavy cover is next to the body, one may be too warm with it and too cold without it, while the thin cover next to the body might be just right. In a cold room a thin mattress may need a blanket over it under the sleeper to equalize warmth above and below.

Mattresses should be turned over or have the ends reversed frequently to equalize wear and promote airing. Mattresses can be bought that are made in two parts, one part being of equal length and width. This provides more possible changes of position.

A mattress need not be discarded when it becomes hard or lumpy from use. The padding can be reworked to produce a mattress practically as good as new. This applies to inner-spring mattresses as well as to those made entirely of cotton or hair. Any mattress factory can do the work, and some furniture stores offer such service.

Feather beds have pretty well gone out of use in America. They are too soft for easy change of position, and in warm weather they add greatly to the discomfort from heat. A feather mattress tightly sewed is good where a soft mattress or only a pad is desired.

Sponge rubber mattresses are now being widely used. When thin enough and firm enough they are satisfactory. If used on springs, the springs should be quite firm, otherwise the rubber tends to wrap around the body, increasing heat and making turning difficult. Rubber mattresses have the great advantage that they do not pack down or become lumpy in use.

When buying a mattress or mattress and springs it should always be tested by lying on it and especially by turning in different positions. Discomfort in any position will indicate that it is probably too hard, while if it is too soft turning will be difficult.

Beds and mattresses are now made in standard widths and lengths which are quite satisfactory except for extra tall people. The standard length of six feet and four inches is satisfactory for the people who are not taller than five feet and ten inches, thus giving a spare length of six inches, which is considered a necessary minimum for comfort. Any metalworking shop can lengthen bed rails by cutting them and inserting a short length of extra rail. These extra pieces should be inserted near the foot of the bed where they are subject to less strain. Mattresses of extra length are not usually carried in stock, so must usually be made to special order. For economy, pillows, or any kind of pad, can be placed at the foot end of the mattress to take up the extra space. Lengthening springs is not usually practicable, but a board of suitable width bolted to the top of the spring at the foot is usually satisfactory. This matter of extra length may seem troublesome or expensive, but it is an investment that will bring big dividends in comfort and sleep.

Your Head on the Pillow. Pillows are an essential part of the bed, but they seldom get the attention they deserve. When men slept on the ground in their caves with only a bear skin under them, an extra skin was probably folded for an extra cushion under the thinly covered bones of the head. Many centuries later when feather beds and mattresses began to be used the extra head cushion was found to be still desirable in order to keep the neck in a comfortable position. In recent years it has begun to be realized that pillows, while still supplying comfort, can and should be used for an even more important purpose, that of protecting the body from harmful strains and pressures during sleep. But if they are to serve this purpose effectively, pillows cannot be limited to one size or shape, or to one degree of softness or firmness. They must be carefully adapted to the requirements of the different positions assumed by the body during sleep, to the different parts of the body which they are to protect, and to the weight and age of the sleeper.

At first thought this may seem like attaching undue importance to pillows. But when we realize that much inability to sleep, or interrupted and unrestful sleep, with resulting unfitness for work, is due to the lack of completely comfortable and relaxing positions of the body while in bed, and even more important, *when we learn that many stubborn and seemingly mysterious cases of arthritis, neuritis, bursitis, etc., owe their beginning and their stubborn persistence to strains and pressures produced by improper positions maintained unconsciously during sleep, we see that proper variety and proper use of pillows is a small price to pay for relief from these handicaps.*

Pillows most commonly are used merely as a support for the head, so we will consider this use first. In this use they make two worthwhile contributions to restful sleep. Because of their softness they support the weight of the head without an uncomfortable concentration of pressure at any one point. Concentrated pressure would require frequent movement of the head for its relief and in this way disturb sleep. A second and more important function of a head pillow is to maintain the neck in proper alignment with the body.

Since the head is of smaller diameter than the body, it must be out of alignment with the body on three sides. Standing with either side or the back against a wall, the head can be made to touch the wall only by distortion of the neck, slight at the back, but severe at the sides. So a pillow would be needed when sleeping in any position except face-down. This position is seldom used, because it interferes with breathing both by obstructing the flow of air to the nose and by hindering the expansion of the chest and abdomen.

Your Sensitive Neck and What to Do About It.   The muscles of the neck are one of the most sensitive and highly organized groups in the body. Their constant use in positioning the eyes makes it necessary that they be highly responsive, requiring many and delicate nerve connections with the brain. When they are forced into strained positions they send a stream of complaining nerve impulses to the brain, seriously disturbing or even preventing sleep. But a still more serious effect is that when these muscles are held under strain through successive nights the muscles and their nerves are likely to develop a chronic inflammation with soreness and twinges of pain. Since there is no surface indication of injury, this condition is likely to be diagnosed and treated as rheumatism or neuritis. But with nothing done to remove the cause, the relief obtained, if any, can be only temporary.

Another danger from a cramped position of the neck is that it may cause compression of the carotid arteries which carry blood to the head and the brain. These arteries are named from the Greek word, *karos,* stupor, because it was found that compressing them would produce mental dullness. Recent studies have shown that during sleep the brain's arteries are normally dilated and carry a larger supply of blood to the brain than is required to maintain the activities of the brain during wakefulness. Consequently it seems likely that reduction of the blood supply during sleep would hinder the rest and recuperation of the brain, which apparently is the main reason why we need to sleep.

To maintain a normal position of the head and neck during sleep, the present writer uses three pillows, two rather soft and flat, the third flat but very firm. When sleeping on his back one soft pillow is used. On his side a soft pillow is used on top of the firm one, the two raising his head enough above the mattress to keep his neck in line with his spine. The advantage of the two pillows over one large soft one is that sufficient height is secured without having the head sink deeply into the pillow, which would cause over-heating and make a change of position more difficult. A dislocation of his right shoulder several years ago which was diagnosed and treated·as rheumatism left that shoulder so sensitive to pressure that sleeping on his right side is not possible. With the double pillow near one side of the bed and the single soft one adjoining it, shifting to the low pillow when turning to the back position is so easy that it is often done without complete awakening.

Recently after sleeping two or three months on a new and firmer mattress, mostly on his left side, the author began to have pains in his left shoulder, such as ordinarily can be attributed to arthritis or bursitis. Suspecting that the pains might be due simply to too much pressure of the shoulder against the new firm mattress, a pad about twelve by eighteen inches was placed under his body just below the armpit, in this way taking his body's weight off the painful shoulder. Without further treatment the pains disappeared within a few days and have not returned. The pad used was made by folding a cotton blanket and covering it with a small pillowcase. Naturally after this experience the pad was not discarded but was kept as a permanent part of the bed's equipment, just as the head pillows are.

With the use of this under-arm pad the left side position became so entirely comfortable that the back position was used very little. The result was that after a short time twinges of pain began to occur in the upper shoulder, the right one which had been made sensitive by a previous injury. The right arm had been allowed to rest on the mattress in front of the body, and upon consideration it seemed likely that the weight of the arm had pulled the shoulder joint down into an irritating position. A plump pillow was then placed on the mattress in front of the body so that it would hold the right forearm almost level with the shoulder. The pains disappeared promptly and have not returned. This pillow, too, has been retained in permanent use.

Pillows of many kinds are sold in Norman Dine's Sleep Shop in New York, but pillows of almost any shape, thickness, or softness can be made with little trouble by starting with ordinary pillow ticks filled either with feathers or with shredded sponge rubber. A very flat, soft pillow can be made by removing part of the filling. A firmer pillow can be made by adding to the filler, or simply by shaking the filler toward one end of the case and doubling the empty end back and fastening it with safety pins. By shaking the filler into one half of the tick and folding the other half over, a very plump and almost square pillow can be made. If the filler is shaken to one edge of the tick, a long, narrow, firm pillow will result. As a support for the head, sponge rubber is to be preferred to feathers because it is not subject to packing and has no odor or allergic effect. Shredded rubber is better than a one-piece block because it lends itself to change as needed.

Don't Give Up the Pillow

Sleeping without pillows cannot be recommended except for very young children. When attempted it is apt to lead to a habit of sleeping with the head on the arm or on the hands. Both these positions put pressure on nerves and blood vessels which may cause serious disorders. Injuries which occur at nerve endings are the only ones that can be properly located by the brain. Injury to a nerve along its course may seem to be located some distance away along the course of the nerve. This makes nerve-pressure pains very deceptive and likely to lead to useless treatment. The only safe course is not to maintain any position very long at a time if it can cause pressure on a nerve. In sleep one is likely to be unconscious of the slight local discomfort caused by the pressure and so to maintain and repeat it until serious pain is felt, pain which unfortunately may not point to the real source of the trouble.

Summary: More Pillows for Old Bones

As people get older their bones seem to get sharper and the cushion of flesh and skin becomes less effective. For example, when one knee is placed upon the other, which is the most natural position when sleeping on the side, the lumps of bone on one knee joint may punch sharply into the corresponding lumps of the other knee. To overcome this discomfort a small, soft cushion should be placed between the knees. This cushion can be made by folding a wool scarf and placing it in a small pillowcase.

Dr. David Fink, in discussing relaxation as an aid to sleep, recommends the use of pillows under the arms and legs. A single long pillow can be so placed as to support both knees, while a separate pillow is used under each forearm. The arms and legs afford more complete relaxation to the muscles when they are slightly bent, and these pillows overcome the severely straight position which is necessary when one lies on his back with his arms and legs resting directly on the mattress. And it must be remembered that muscles when fully relaxed are sending the minimum number of nerve impulses to the brain and so are offering the least hindrance to sleep.

A very thorough discussion of beds, pillows, and positions of the body during sleep will be found in the book *Sleep, the Secret of Greater Power and Achievement,* by Ray Giles.

9. How to ventilate
your bedroom

How Many Barrels of Air Does Your Bedroom Need?

Many statements have been made about the urgent need for ventilation in the bedroom, but few verifiable measurements have been given in support of these assertions. One author states that "twenty-five barrels" of air are breathed by a sleeper during eight hours of sleep, and then argues from this that open windows are an absolute necessity. Let us see how well this argument stands up.

The average person when at rest breathes sixteen times a minute, inhaling approximately a pint of air at each breath. This means he uses air at the rate of two gallons a minute, or 120 gallons an hour. The amount of air a person breathes is considerably reduced during sleep, but to make allowances for all variations we will overlook this reduction and make our calculations on the basis of breathing when awake. In eight hours at 120 gallons an hour our sleeper would breathe 960 gallons of air. Most barrels in common use hold 50 gallons or thereabouts. So we will allow 50 gallons to the barrel, and divide 960 by 50 to get the number of barrels. This gives us for the night's breathing just over 19 barrels.

But let us say that our sleeper is a heavy breather and does actually breathe 25 barrels during the night, would this exhaust the air in a room? An average room is something like 12 by 14 feet, with an eight-foot ceiling. Multiplication of these dimensions gives 1344 cubic feet, or allowing space for furniture we will say that our room contains 1300 cubic feet of air. A cubic foot is almost exactly seven and a half gallons. Multiplying our cubic feet by seven and a half we get 9,750 gallons as the total amount of air which the room contains. This we divide by 50 to find that the room holds 195 barrels. From this we see at once that a sleeper in breathing 25 barrels would make only a small beginning on the air in the average-sized room. *Two people sleeping in the room could breathe hardly more than a fourth of the air in the room in eight hours.*

And this is only part of the story. In our calculations we have assumed that the room is airtight. As a matter of fact, even in the closest room and with no wind pressure, there is a constant seepage of air around doors and windows and through the walls. Under ordinary conditions this probably supplies in the course of the night much more air than a sleeper breathes, in poorly built houses several times as much. A moderate wind greatly increases this change of air.

A further fact that must not be overlooked is that even when we have breathed a certain portion of air, we have not used up all its oxygen. Approximately 20 per cent, or one-fifth, of the air is oxygen. After it is breathed it still contains about 16 per cent of oxygen. If a person were in an airtight room he would have to breathe all the air at least twice before the lack of oxygen would cause him any serious discomfort, and even then it would not have reached the danger point. Only 10 or 12 per cent of oxygen is needed to support life.

But how about the carbon dioxide that our lungs throw off? Doesn't that make ventilation necessary? Air before it is breathed contains only a small fraction of one per cent of carbon dioxide. When it is breathed it takes up a slightly smaller amount of carbon dioxide than it loses of oxygen, that is, of its entire volume about four per cent of oxygen has been lost and about three and one-half per cent of carbon dioxide has been taken up. No effect will be noticed from breathing this air except a moderate increase in the rate of breathing. Because of its effect in stimulating breathing, air or oxygen which contains seven or eight per cent of carbon dioxide is often used to speed revival of people who have lost consciousness in drowning or suffocation. So far as any harmful effect is concerned, air could be breathed a second and even a third time and still have a wide margin of safety in its carbon dioxide content. Only when carbon dioxide is increased to 25 per cent, one fourth of the entire volume of the air, will it cause fainting, and it must go higher still before its effect becomes dangerous. So we see that there is an even wider margin of safety from the accumulation of carbon dioxide than from the reduction of oxygen.

When the Air Is "Stuffy"

The increased use of air conditioning is helping us to realize that it is temperature and humidity we must watch, both for comfort and for health. When air becomes what we call stuffy it is almost invariably due to an increase of temperature or humidity, or both, and almost never due to a lack of oxygen or to an excess of carbon dioxide. This has been effectively demonstrated by a simple experiment using a telephone booth with a head opening in it. This opening was closed and the booth used until the air inside became stuffy enough to cause headache and nausea. At this point an experimenter who was outside thrust his head through the opening so that he must breathe the air inside. With his body in the relatively cool and dry air outside, simply breathing the stuffy air inside the booth did not cause him any discomfort. The person inside the booth was affected by the accumulation of heat and moisture, which prevented proper cooling of his body by evaporation of perspiration from his skin, and not by the air in his lungs.

The absence of any effect upon the lungs from increased heat and moisture is not difficult to understand when we recall that air passing from the nostrils to the lungs is raised to a temperature well above that of a stuffy room, and that its content of moisture reaches almost the saturation point. Consequently any ordinary increase of heat and moisture in the air breathed cannot perceptibly change the air inside the lungs. And it will be recalled that, as stated previously, the entire volume of air in the booth could be breathed two or three times before the lack of oxygen or the increase of carbon dioxide could cause serious discomfort. In view of these facts the outcome of the experiment in the telephone booth is easy to understand. What we call stuffiness of the air actually produces its effect through the skin. Hot and humid air do not take up the heat and moisture of the skin rapidly enough for comfort. When the air is in motion the discomfort caused by heat and humidity is much less, since moving air carries both heat and moisture away from the body much more rapidly. This is the reason why the air from a fan always feels cool and gives relief from heat, though its temperature and its moisture content have not been changed.

Facts such as these make it clear that in ventilating our bedrooms we should aim at comfort, through control of heat, humidity, and air movement, and that any danger from lack of oxygen or excess of carbon dioxide is largely imaginary. Air movement must be properly controlled to avoid creating a draft. In cold weather this can result from even a partial opening of a window.

Watch Out for Carbon Monoxide

The gas that is dangerous in bedrooms is carbon monoxide, one atom of carbon combined with one atom of oxygen. This gas is a product of incomplete burning of fuels, such as gas, oil, coal and wood, and it should cause very serious concern if there is any source from which it could reach the bedroom.

When any fuel containing carbon is burned it is possible for the carbon to combine with the oxygen of the air in two proportions. When there is an ample supply of air, each atom of carbon takes up two atoms of oxygen from the air, the product being carbon dioxide, a gas which is not poisonous, and except in extremely high concentrations is entirely harmless. But when a stove or furnace has a reduced air supply each atom of carbon may combine with only one atom of oxygen, and so produce carbon monoxide, a gas which is a deadly poison. Only a small fraction of one per cent in the air will cause death. This gas has no color and no odor, so that it cannot be seen or smelled, and usually there is no bodily discomfort to warn of its presence. *Persons sleeping in a bedroom where the air contains as much as one fourth of one per cent of carbon monoxide will not live through the night.*

Any fire burning in a bedroom may become a source of carbon monoxide, but oil and gas heaters are the most likely sources, because in many cases they are used without flues or vent pipes to carry away the gases that are produced by the flames. Unless it has an outside vent, no heater should ever be left burning in a bedroom. In fact, such a heater should not be used in any room except for a short time. Its use in a bathroom is especially dangerous because of the small size of the room.

Heaters with smoke pipes, including those burning coal and wood, may be dangerous sources of carbon monoxide if there is a damper in the pipe. Such a damper produces its effects in two ways. First it reduces the amount of air drawn into the fire, in this way reducing the supply of oxygen so that more carbon monoxide is formed, and in the second place it cuts off the outlet for the gases formed, so that they are forced out at all the joints of the heater into the air of the room. The draft in a heater should always be controlled by regulating the intake of air and not by reducing the outlet of the gases produced by the fire.

Furnaces located in small rooms or closets and circulating warm air by means of a fan are especially dangerous when they have draft diverters in the smoke pipe. If by any chance the air circulation intake from the rooms of the house to the furnace room is cut off or clogged, then the gases from the smoke pipe will be sucked out of the diverter by the circulating fan and sent through the house.

A furnace in the basement may introduce a dangerous amount of carbon monoxide into a bedroom if it is of either the hot air or forced warm air type. A furnace controlled by a damper in the smoke pipe may leak gases from the fire into the air jacket, and from this they are carried to the various rooms of the house. Such a furnace when fired by a stoker is dangerous if the blow of the stoker fan is too strong for the size of the smoke pipe or if the smoke pipe is clogged with soot, so that a pressure is built up in the firebox by the blow from the fan. The air flow from the fan to the fire should be adjusted so that no smoke comes out of the furnace door when it is open and the fan is running. With this adjustment all gases rising from the fire are carried into the chimney. The hopper of a stoker should be kept tightly closed except while it is being filled. Otherwise air pressure from the fan may force gases from the fire back through the worm pipe which feeds the coal, and they will then escape from the hopper into the furnace room and seep throughout the house. Joints and openings of the coal feed pipe if not gas tight may leak carbon monoxide into the furnace room.

Symptoms and Effects of Carbon Monoxide Poisoning

Very small traces of carbon monoxide in the air, if breathed continuously or repeatedly, can produce serious results which show up later on. Not even the smallest trace of this gas should be considered safe. A few people develop a certain amount of tolerance to this gas, but in most people any tolerance they may have at the start is gradually lost, and the effects slowly become worse. The effects often are not felt immediately. They may include dizziness, drowsiness, nausea, irritability, persistent headache, and predisposition to accidents.

Carbon monoxide produces its effects by interfering with the oxygen supply of the body and especially of the brain. Oxygen is carried from the lungs to various parts of the body by the red cells of the blood. Carbon monoxide has what chemists call a great affinity for these red cells, more than two hundred times the affinity that oxygen has. When the red cells are carrying carbon monoxide they cannot carry oxygen. So if the air breathed contains only one two-hundredth as much carbon monoxide as it does of oxygen, the carbon monoxide will still take over half of the red cells of the blood. This means that if the air breathed contains only one-tenth of one per cent of carbon monoxide as against its twenty per cent of oxygen, the blood will be able to carry only half its normal amount of oxygen. Since the brain cannot maintain consciousness when the oxygen of the blood falls below one-third of its normal content, the remaining margin of safety would be very small. Any weakness of the lungs or any deficiency in the blood circulation, or any exertion calling for the use of more oxygen, would be likely to bring on the unconsciousness which we call fainting.

First Aid to Victims

When a person has absorbed enough carbon monoxide to cause fainting, the important and urgent thing to do is to remove him from the room which contains the poisoned air in order to stop his absorption of the poison. If his breathing has stopped, he must be given artificial respiration immediately, continuing until natural breathing starts. Hospitals and rescue squads have tanks of oxygen containing a small percentage of carbon dioxide. This mixture, if available, should be breathed during artificial respiration and for a short time afterward until deep natural breathing has returned. The high percentage of oxygen in this mixture tends to displace the carbon monoxide, and equally important, the carbon dioxide acts as a stimulant to the respiratory center of the brain. The resulting increase in breathing passes the oxygen through the lungs much more rapidly and causes a much more rapid washing out of the carbon monoxide from the blood.

If carbon dioxide from tanks is not available, holding a paper bag over the patient's nose and mouth during a few breaths will aid in starting natural breathing or in deepening it, because the patient's breath, which he rebreathes from the bag, contains a sufficient amount of carbon dioxide to act as a stimulant of the respiratory center of the brain. The only cure for carbon monoxide poisoning is to wash the poisonous gas out of the blood by breathing uncontaminated air promptly and rapidly. If this is not done without delay, the brain will be permanently damaged by lack of oxygen.

Summary: Our Body's Wonderful Chemistry

Though most of the body's heat and energy comes from combining carbon with oxygen, no carbon monoxide is ever produced. This is a mark of the high efficiency of the body's chemistry, for more heat or energy is produced when every atom of carbon is combined with its full quota of two atoms of oxygen. This means safety, too, as well as efficiency, since instead of the poisonous carbon monoxide, carbon dioxide is produced, which is completely harmless and is also highly useful as a regulator of body processes.

Man-made devices for producing heat and energy are usually less efficient, and are often highly dangerous. Man's widely used device for producing power, the gasoline engine, in which a carbon-containing gas is burned in a tightly closed cylinder, is a prolific producer of carbon monoxide, especially when the carburetor is improperly adjusted or when the choke is being used causing a reduction of the normal air supply. Many deaths are caused every year by the operation of such engines in closed rooms.

The great importance of carbon monoxide as a factor to be considered in ventilation is well illustrated by the fact that the engineers who built the tunnel under the East River from New York to Brooklyn have based their control of ventilation in the tunnel entirely on the percentage of carbon monoxide in the air. Detectors are placed at intervals along the tunnel and their readings are registered in the control room. No danger is anticipated from the lack of oxygen or excess of carbon dioxide as long as the carbon monoxide is held within safe limits.

10. Simple exercises
to promote sleep

Workout For Sleep

That muscular fatigue tends to bring on sleep must be evident to everyone from personal experience. Various methods of exercising as a preparation for sleep have been recommended, and if one's usual activities do not call for much physical exertion, some muscular exercise may prove very helpful.

For those who wish to try exercise before retiring, the following series of body movements will be found convenient and effective. Proved and improved by the author over a period of many years, these movements are suited for limbering up the joints, loosening the muscles, and stimulating the circulation, as well as for producing fatigue. They do not require any special equipment, and all are made in the standing position except the massage of the feet. They give the body a quick workout from top to toe, and the whole series requires hardly more than ten minutes. The movements are simple and the sequence logical, so that no difficulty will be experienced in remembering them or in learning to do them correctly.

Workout For Waking Up

These movements are also used by the author as an eye-opener on arising in the morning in order to throw off more quickly the sluggishness which is always carried over somewhat from sleep. The movements are vigorous enough to raise the body temperature and to quicken respiration and circulation, but not so violent as to cause straining of any muscle.

In beginning these exercises a person in ordinary health can very well start by repeating each movement five times. After one becomes accustomed to the movements it is better not to make any attempt at counting them but to do each one until a slight sensation of fatigue is felt. This gives an easy and flexible means of adjusting each movement to the strength of its particular set of muscles, and also to the general vigor of the body at the time. An effort should be made to extend gradually each movement somewhat further as the muscles and joints begin to loosen up with practice.

In case one wishes to tire himself out thoroughly, a good plan is to repeat the whole series of movements several times, or until the desired degree of fatigue is obtained.

In executing these movements attention should be given to keeping all the muscles relaxed except those actually concerned in the movement being used. Special effort should be made to avoid holding any part of the body stiff or rigidly fixed. This muscular looseness is a good condition to cultivate in all one's activities throughout the day. It is essentially the same thing that Dr. Edmund Jacobson has urged under the title of "differential relaxation" and that W. H. Miller speaks of as "unlocking the muscles."

No advantage will be gained by trying to time the breathing in unison with the various movements. The breaths should be full and taken only as rapidly as may be demanded by the exertion of each movement.

Exercises To Do Five Times Each.   The movements begin with the feet and work upward to the head. They are best taken in light clothing, or in the nude if in a warm room. During the foot and leg movements, except No. 4, the body should be steadied by placing one hand on a table or other support.

First Movement: Stand with the heels six or eight inches apart, toes turned slightly outward. Raise and lower the weight of the body on the toes. *This movement will strengthen the arches and loosen the ankles.*

Second Movement: Same position as first movement. Now lift the toes from the floor as far as possible, allowing the weight of the body to rest on the heels. *This movement helps further to loosen the ankles and brings in an opposite and little-used set of muscles.*

Third Movement: Stand with the heels ten or twelve inches apart and the feet nearly parallel. Roll the feet from the ankles, first to the right, then to the left, turning the feet on the sides as far as possible. This will require a partial bending of the knees also. *This movement is an excellent ankle loosener and will strengthen the muscles which guard against accidental turning of the ankles in walking.*

Fourth Movement: Stand erect, with the arms hanging straight down from the shoulders. First bend and then straighten the knees, so that the arms move straight up and down. The finger tips should come down to the ankles without bending the back. *This movement lifts the body with the same muscles which a trained workman uses in lifting a heavy weight. The strong muscles of the legs do the work, thus relieving the back.*

Fifth Movement: Stand on the left foot and lift the right hip so that the right foot will clear the floor, then swing the right foot forward and backward as far as possible.

Sixth Movement: Same as the fifth movement but standing on the right foot and swinging the left foot.

Seventh Movement: Stand so that the support used for steadying the body is directly in front, but keep the body erect. Lift the right hip and swing the right foot across in front of the body, back and forth, bringing the foot as far up as possible on each side.

Eighth Movement: Same as the seventh but swinging the left foot.

Ninth Movement: Stand with the heels twelve to fifteen inches apart. Place the hands on the hips and bend the trunk well forward. Allow the knees to bend very slightly. Swing the trunk to the right and then on around in a circle, bending as far to the sides and back as possible. The hips should swing in unison with the trunk but outward in the opposite direction, in order to maintain the body balance. *This movement involves not only the muscles and joints of the hips and lower back but also of the knees and ankles.*

Tenth Movement: Same as the ninth but swinging the trunk in the opposite direction.

Movements five to ten will thoroughly loosen the joints and muscles of the hips and of the lower back and abdomen.

Eleventh Movement: Place the backs of the hands against the spine and with strong pressure on them move them down to the hips and then up the spine as far as possible, repeating the movement until fatigue is felt in the arms. The hands should move a short distance from side to side as well as up and down, using the first finger joints to reach into depressions alongside the spine. *In addition to massaging the spinal muscles, this movement exercises the muscles which move the wrists backward and brings into play other seldom-used muscles of the arms.*

Twelfth Movement: Holding the arms straight out in front and keeping them together swing them first right then left with considerable force, so that they pull the shoulders around toward the rear as far as possible. The head, too, should be turned with the shoulders so that an object directly to the rear can be seen from both the right and the left extreme positions. *This movement gives the spine a thorough twisting to loosen up the joints between the vertebrae. It is also splendid exercise for the shoulders and the neck.* This movement requires exhaling strongly at the end of each swing, when both chest and abdomen are strongly compressed, then inhaling as the next swing starts.

Thirteenth Movement: Swing both arms in circles from the shoulders, up in front, all the way back, down, forward; up, back, down, forward; and so on.

Fourteenth Movement: Same as the thirteenth except circling in the opposite direction; down in front, back, up, forward. *These two movements keep the shoulder joints loose and flexible, and help to guard against arthritis of the shoulder.*

Fifteenth Movement: (For optional use if desired to develop the biceps and triceps muscles, the muscles which bend and straighten the elbows.) Place the left hand limply against the breastbone. Extend the right arm upward, outward, and slightly forward to full length. Then bend the arm at the elbow by contracting the biceps until the hand rests loosely against the breastbone, making this movement slowly and opposing it strongly with the triceps. Next, straighten the arm slowly by contracting the triceps while opposing it with the biceps. Now return the right arm to the breastbone and repeat the movements with the left arm, alternating the arms until a slight degree of fatigue is felt. During both movements the hands must remain completely relaxed and unaffected by the contraction of the large arm muscles.

Besides developing the biceps and triceps, these movements give training in keeping some muscles relaxed while putting forth effort with others. They also illustrate a principle very widely used in exercise systems, the resisting of one muscle or set of muscles with another.

Sixteenth Movement: Stand with the heels well apart. Place the hands together over the head so that the fingers cross at the knuckles and the tips of the fingers and thumbs touch the scalp. With heavy pressure on the scalp and a strong effort of the arms against resistance of the neck, pull the head forward, then to the right, and on around in a circle. The head should be pulled down as far as possible at every point as it swings around. The hips and knees should be flexible and should swing in an opposite direction to the swing of the head in order to keep the body in balance. The hands should be allowed to slide with the pull on the head, in this way giving the scalp a thorough massage.

Seventeenth Movement: This movement is the same as the sixteenth except that the head is circled in the opposite direction.

These last two movements are very important. When properly executed they produce a rhythmic swing of the entire body from the ankles upward, much like that of a good golf stroke, though with a much wider inclusion of muscles. The resulting massage of

*the scalp will improve the circulation of the blood to feed the hair,
which is believed by many to delay baldness. The twisting of the
neck vertebrae will help to prevent the type of nerve pressure that
sometimes causes a neuritis of the arm.*

Eighteenth Movement: This is a rub-down of the entire body with
the open hands, beginning with the arms and working down the
trunk and legs to the ankles, then working back up to the arms,
including on the way up a vigorous massage of the calves of the
legs and the muscles at the back of the thighs together with a
thorough kneading of the abdomen. When the weather is hot and
the body perspiring the hands should be covered with a towel or with
massage mits. *This friction and kneading stimulate and permanently improve the circulation of the blood and in this way tend to
prevent cramps in the muscles, which often interfere with the sleep
of persons past middle age. This massage affords also an excellent
work-out for the muscles of the hands and arms.*

Nineteenth Movement: This movement is really an extension of
the rub-down, and is used while putting on the socks or stockings.
It gives a thorough massage of the feet. Cross the left foot over
the right knee, draw a sock or stocking partly over the right hand,
and with this covered hand give the foot a thorough rubbing and
twisting, then put the sock on the foot and massage the foot again,
working this time with both hands.

Twentieth Movement: This movement is the same as the nineteenth
except that massage is applied to the right foot over the left knee.

*These last two movements are important in giving the circulation
in the feet a much-needed stimulus.* Because our feet are usually
encased in close-fitting and rather stiff shoes, and because they are
at a distance from the heart and in standing and sitting are much
lower than the heart, the circulation is apt to become sluggish.
This is especially true when one position is maintained for some
time, for then the blood in the veins is not forced onward by movements of the muscles. Massage by pressure on the veins speeds
the return of blood to the heart, thus clearing the way for a fresh
supply to flow in from the arteries. Some authorities recommend

massaging the feet whenever they become cold, considering that warming them with a fresh flow of blood is much better than using artificial heat.

Summary: Mainly on Walking

Many writers recommend walking as a splendid exercise to use as a preparation for sleep. It has the advantages of not requiring other persons to make up a team, of being always available, of being perfectly adaptable to the limits of one's time and strength, and also, since it requires little light, of being available in the evening when the majority of us have most leisure.

While there are many who recommend walking, there are few who tell how walking should be done. At most one finds advice that he should include occupation for the mind, such as pleasant conversation, or if alone the observation of wildlife or plants. Little or nothing is said about the physical or mechanical side of walking. Yet this, too, is important. Walking can be highly effective in loosening up the whole muscular and skeletal mechanism of the body if it is properly done.

Walk and Roll. The author vividly recalls a walk which took him through the woods with a Boy Scout executive. He swung along with two heavy suitcases apparently without effort while I with some lighter packages struggled to keep up with him. Afterward I frequently tried to imitate his rolling gait, but I could never quite get it until one day when going down a slight slope on my way into town I saw a long, gangling mountaineer leaning against a telephone pole a short distance ahead of me. Just before I reached him he detached himself from the pole and started off down the sidewalk in front of me. His gait was such a perfect roll that for a moment I felt like rubbing my eyes to make sure that it was a man and not a big wheel that I was watching. Every joint in his body seemed to be loose, and he swung from one foot to the other with hardly more apparent effort than a wheel would make in rolling. Keeping that picture in mind, with further practice I was finally able to gain a fair approximation of the scout executive's gait.

One day I approached a fellow teacher and said abruptly, "Professor Blank, do you know how to walk?" The question apparently seemed to him too preposterous for an immediate answer, so I continued, "Can you walk like this?" at the same time turning away from him and putting on my best imitation of the mountaineer's roll. Turning back to him 1 repeated, "Can you walk like that?" Looking at me with a somewhat scandalized expression he said, "Perhaps I *could,* but some consideration must be given to dignity."

The point I wish to make is that if you want to get the most benefit from your walking exercise you should endeavor to acquire the mountaineer's loose-jointed roll, and not give too much thought to your dignity. You should swing easily from one foot to the other with a motion something like that of skating. Imagine yourself rolling like a wheel with a big soft tire on it, instead of jolting over the ground like a wheel without even a rim, just bumping along on the ends of the spokes. The shocks of such jerky walking are a tax on the spine, while the rhythmic swing of a proper gait serves as a tonic to the whole body. A walk that combines spring with roll produces refreshment with a minimum of fatigue.

Competitive games shortly before retiring, whether the competition is physical or mental, are not recommended as a preparation for sleep. They offer the temptation to stay up beyond normal bedtime, and they are likely to leave both body and mind in a highly stimulated and excited state which will seriously delay the coming of sleep. Games that produce muscular fatigue, if played in the afternoon or in the early part of the evening, may be very helpful in bringing normal sleep.

11. How to attain
relaxation without
a "sleep start"

Three Kinds of Relaxation

Among the many aids to sleep, the one emphasized by the greatest number of writers is relaxation, meaning primarily or exclusively relaxation of the voluntary muscles, the muscles that we use in our purposeful movements. In spite of widespread advocacy, however, relaxation as a means of bringing sleep does not seem to have gained very wide adoption. Ray Giles in his book on sleep gives reports he received from prominent people in all parts of the country when he inquired what they did to lure sleep. The reports show that not one in twenty used relaxation. Of course these people have read the claims made for relaxation, and probably many of them have tried it, but found it ineffective or for some reason unsatisfactory.

The term relaxation has been used with three quite different meanings. Formerly it was much used to mean recreation or amusement, or any release from work or the cares of life. In this sense it applies almost entirely to the mind. A second meaning now much in use implies a sort of philosophy of life, living in a take-it-easy, don't-get-excited frame of mind. But this idea is applied to the body also, and means getting rid of all unnecessary or unconscious muscular tension. This philosophical meaning of relaxation has been emphasized by various writers, and as an art of living to be learned it is of great value. In a third use the term relaxation is limited entirely to the voluntary muscles. It is this third meaning that is most in use by writers on sleep.

The author solved his own problem of wakefulness without giving any thought to relaxation. He did not even suspect at that time that relaxation played any part in bringing sleep. Only afterward did he learn that he had been using without knowing it what he now believes to be the most effective of all means of relaxing the muscles. And he also believes now that it was a decided advantage not to give conscious attention to his muscles. Impulses from the brain to the voluntary muscles can produce only one effect, contraction. No nerves have been found which can carry voluntary impulses of relaxation. Such impulses are not needed, for when contraction impulses stop, the muscles relax of themselves, unconsciously. Attempts to relax the muscles by conscious effort are usually baffling and discouraging, being in fact likely to produce contraction rather than relaxation.

Voluntary contraction of the muscles as it occurs in bodily activity has long been known as the most certain means of preventing sleep. But unconscious muscular contraction has no such prohibitive effect on sleep. A recent scientific study of the measurable characteristics of sleep failed to show any correspondence between the degree of relaxation found in the muscles and the depth of sleep as indicated by the electroencephalograph, now recognized as the best means of measuring the depth of sleep. This study has made it clear that complete relaxation of muscle tonus or other unconsciously maintained contraction of the muscles is not a necessary preparation for sleep. That complete relaxation adds to the restfulness of sleep seems likely, but that it is not a necessary condition of sound sleep is certain.

Jacobson: Stop Contracting

Among advocates of muscular relaxation as a means of inducing sleep Dr. Edmund Jacobson of Chicago seems best known. His ideas have been adopted, with variations, by other writers on sleep. The physiological and psychological basis of the Jacobson system is the habit common among persons doing mental work of unconsciously maintaining some groups of their muscles in a continuous state of contraction. This habit can become so fixed that the contraction persists after work stops, and even continues during sleep. Dr. Jacobson's plan is to try to locate these groups of unconsciously contracting muscles, and then to break the habit of contraction. Because the contraction has become automatic, this is not easy, but takes effort and practice, and usually requires many hours of training under Dr. Jacobson's personal supervision, because he is not content merely to break the faulty habit, but insists on an extreme degree of relaxation which will eliminate even the reflex muscle tonus.

Dr. Jacobson strongly advises against the practices of the Yogi, but when he undertakes to remove muscle tonus, which normally is under reflex control, he is actually entering the same obscure realm which has been exploited by the Yogi for centuries past. After years of training the Yogi are able to make their breathing imperceptible, greatly slow their heart action, and even reduce their body temperature, reaching almost the state of a hibernating animal. Physiologists studying the exploits of the Yogi have performed equally strange feats, learning by long practice to make their hair stand on end, or even to make their pancreatic glands secrete more insulin. These feats, as well as the achievements of Dr. Jacobson's patients, have amply proved that with sufficient time and effort it is possible to gain some voluntary control of muscle action which normally is under unconscious reflex control. But the practical question which concerns us here is whether it is necessary or desirable to resort to such extreme measures in order to bring sleep.

Dr. Jacobson claims that no means other than muscular relaxation are used in his method of inducing sleep, but other aids are in fact present and active in his procedures. He admits that in some instances "repose" seems to be slightly aided by diverting the patient's attention away from his worries and directing it to the state of his muscles, but he considers this diversion to be merely a desirable by-product of relaxation. He specifically states that he does not use controlled breathing. Yet he notes that when the muscles of the chest are relaxed, respiration becomes slower and shallower. This, of course, reduces the volume of air breathed and increases the percentage of carbon dioxide in the blood. As pointed out in chapter 16 this is an excellent substitute for sleeping pills. Added to this is the fatigue produced by baffling attempts to obtain voluntary control over reflexly controlled muscles, and fatigue, as we all know, is a very potent aid to sleep. Thus Dr. Jacobson overlooks or discounts three very important aids to sleep —mind diversion, hypnotic action of carbon dioxide, and frustrated fatigue—which might well produce sleep even before any considerable degree of relaxation is reached. In fact, much of the doctor's success in treating nervous tension may quite possibly be due to the fact that his patients, in the course of their efforts to attain extreme relaxation, gain the curative effects of sleep through these unrecognized aids.

Kennedy: Think Black, Breathe Slowly

Another man whose advocacy of relaxation as an aid to sleep has received wide publicity is Mr. Joseph Kennedy of Atlanta. His system shows some marked differences from that of Dr. Jacobson, both in aims and in procedures. Dr. Jacobson says that no effort should be made to stop thinking, but that reliance should be placed entirely on muscle relaxation. Mr. Kennedy says that mental imagery should be obliterated by remembering or imagining absolute black. Dr. Jacobson cautions against any form of breathing control, while Mr. Kennedy makes slowing of the breathing one of his three basic steps in securing relaxation. Dr. Jacobson begins his training with the large muscles and ends with the fine muscles of the eyes and speech. Mr. Kennedy follows the opposite order, starting with the eyes and progressing downward over the body. Dr. Jacobson trains only one group of muscles at a time, spending an hour or more on one group and attempting to obtain complete relaxation of this group before proceeding to another group. Mr. Kennedy's method is to go over the whole body at one session, strongly contracting each group of muscles and then leaving it to relax unconsciously while attention is diverted to another group. Dr. Jacobson does not encourage his clients to expect noticeable results from relaxation until after at least several weeks of training and practice. Mr. Kennedy says that a definite sense of relaxation should be experienced after the first or second period of training. Dr. Jacobson aims at bringing normally involuntary muscle tonus under voluntary control, while Mr. Kennedy attempts as far as possible to bring voluntary muscles under unconscious control, which he claims gives both more complete relaxation for sleep and better muscular coordination in activities. While neither of these two authors makes the definite statement that relaxation and sleep are the same thing, both say unqualifiedly that when complete relaxation is attained, sleep always comes with it. *The present author believes that when properly interpreted this most likely means simply that complete relaxation occurs only in sleep.*

Mr. Kennedy began the teaching of relaxation as a means of improving athletic activities, and its use as an aid to sleep is for him more or less incidental. From this standpoint his procedures are excellent, and in most respects are based on sound physiology. It is unfortunate, though, that he has accepted the old physiological myth that an increase of breathing will increase the amount of oxygen used by the body. It is true, as he says, that most nervous people over-ventilate, breathing too fast and too deeply, thus over-stimulating the metabolic activity of the body. But this is due not to an over-supply of oxygen, as he states, but to the washing of carbon dioxide out of the blood. This leaves the blood more alkaline than it should be, and this alkalinity makes the nerves abnormally excitable and metabolism too rapid. Oxygen supply is little affected by over-breathing, because with normal breathing the blood leaves the lungs almost one hundred per cent saturated with oxygen, so that there is little room for an increase. And the organs of the body make use of oxygen only according to their

D

needs, ordinarily using only a fraction of what the blood carries. Oxygen supply to the muscles is probably the principal limiting factor in strenuous athletic activities, but this is a matter of how much oxygen the blood can carry, and not of any limitation of supply from the air in the lungs. Except in strenuous exertion the oxygen supply carried by the blood is more than ample. Over-breathing does not increase the oxygen in the blood materially, nor does it cause the body to absorb more oxygen from the blood.

A similar error appears in the opposite direction in Mr. Kennedy's discussion of the reduced breathing which he lists as the second of the three "physiological switches" he uses to "turn on" relaxation.

It is true that reduced breathing does slow down nerve function and the functions of the body in general, as Mr. Kennedy says. But this effect is not due to a decrease in the body's oxygen supply. The surplus of oxygen taken into the lungs in ordinary breathing is so great that the moderate reduction in breathing which Mr. Kennedy's instructions call for would still ensure practically 100 per cent saturation of the blood with oxygen. The important effect of the reduced breathing is that it carries less carbon dioxide away from the lungs, leaving a larger content of carbon dioxide in the blood, thus creating a mild respiratory acidosis, and this slows down nerve action.

Mr. Kennedy cites the work of Dr. L. J. Meduna as evidence that carbon dioxide decreases the excitability of the nerve cells in the brain, but he evidently fails to realize that when his clients reduce their breathing the resulting aid to relaxation is due to an increase in the carbon dioxide content of their blood, for immediately following this reference, and a similar one to Dr. William Osler, he again attributes the relaxing effect to a lowered oxygen supply.

Other Views

Short discussions of relaxation as an aid to sleep can be found in the books of various authors. One of the best of these is in

Release from Nervous Tension, by Dr. David Fink. The procedures he recommends are quite similar to those of Dr. Jacobson, but much simplified. He does not consider it necessary to have a physician's instruction or supervision. He estimates that an intelligent adult can teach himself to relax in about ten weeks, and that at the end of three weeks' practice one should have no trouble in falling asleep at night. He, like Dr. Jacobson and Mr. Kennedy, attaches great importance to relaxation of the muscles of the eyes and of speech. He emphasizes relaxation of the chest muscles, accompanied by slowed, quiet, breathing, but fails to note the nerve-quieting effect which this produces through an increase of carbon dioxide in the blood. He says that the most continuous and most effective practice in relaxation is secured while asleep, and that habitual muscle tensions can be lost during sleep, statements which have the present writer's unqualified endorsement. In his more recent book, *Be Your Real Self,* Dr. Fink has somewhat abbreviated his instructions for relaxation and further enumerated its benefits.

Another author meriting mention as an advocate of relaxation and of its use as an aid to sleep is Josephine Rathbone of Columbia University. In her books, *Relaxation* and *Teach Yourself to Relax,* she outlines a number of exercises designed to relax tensions in various parts of the body. Among them she lists some Yoga poses. She quotes Dr. Jacobson's instructions at considerable length, offering them as a means of training the muscles to relax at will. She comments, however, that his technique is extremely hard to master. She approves of controlled breathing, but without mentioning the quieting effect upon the nerves which it produces by accumulating carbon dioxide in the body. Though she gives a list of ten "simple tricks" which can be used as sleep inducers, her main emphasis is not on securing sleep but on overcoming chronic and cumulative fatigue, and she suggests various means of arresting the progress of these conditions before they result in exhaustion and breakdown, adequate sleep being offered as a potent means to this end.

Dr. James Bender in his book, *How to Sleep*, gives an extensive list of relaxing exercises. After his statement that Yoga practices embrace eighty thousand or more methods, exercises, and postures, his list may seem moderate, though it embraces twenty-eight main numbers, many of them with four or more lettered subdivisions. He holds that you can relax muscles after tiring them, and apparently his list of exercises was made with this idea in mind. He makes no effort to eliminate muscle tonus and believes that no one is ever fully relaxed, even in sleep. He specifies that each group of muscles should be contracted five times or more before passing to another group. If fatigue will produce relaxation, and relaxation can be depended on to bring sleep, this method should prove successful. As a practical every-day aid to sleep, however, such a laborious procedure certainly has serious limitations.

All authorities agree that it is only as a result of the most extreme fatigue that a person can sleep while any considerable group of his voluntary muscles is in active contraction. This has been recognized in a very practical way by military commanders for thousands of years. No sentry goes to sleep as long as he obeys his orders to continuously patrol his beat. Both men and animals when preparing for sleep instinctively assume a position which does not require active contraction of the voluntary muscles. Another point on which the best authorities agree, however, is that nothing like complete relaxation is necessary as a preparation for sleep. They hold, in fact, that complete relaxation is seldom attained, even during sleep. Under normal healthy conditions of body and mind as much relaxation of the voluntary muscles as is needed for sleep can be secured merely by stopping voluntary movements while the body is in a position favorable to relaxation. Under such conditions relaxation is not a problem and does not need to be given any special attention. When the nerve impulses that cause muscle contraction are stopped the muscles relax automatically, and the return impulses which they send to the brain are reduced to a point where they do not interfere with the coming of sleep.

When we come to consider involuntary muscular contraction, especially the type of muscular contraction which is responsible for muscle tonus, we find a very significant difference. Relaxation of muscle tonus, it would seem, is neither necessary nor usual as a preparation for sleep. Once sleep has set in, though, most muscular contraction of this type is released automatically. Usually this occurs without the sleeper being aware of it, but it may occur under such conditions as to wake the sleeper. A familiar example of this is the ordinary sleepy nod. *This experience offers convincing proof that it is sleep that brings relaxation, and not the relaxation that brings sleep.* Anyone who has had this experience knows that it was after he had gone to sleep that his neck muscles relaxed and dropped his head, bringing a surprised and, if he was in a public gathering, a shame-faced awakening. Ordinarily the head is held erect by an unconscious tonus in the neck muscles, and it is the release of this tonus by sleep that causes the nod. It would seem that the reason why muscle tonus does not interfere with the approach of sleep is that it can be maintained by reflexes which do not reach the centers of consciousness in the brain.

The "Sleep Start"

In connection with relaxation the familiar "sleep start" requires consideration. This is a sudden muscular contraction, followed by an almost equally sudden relaxation. It usually occurs within the first few minutes after the beginning of sleep, and it commonly affects only a single muscle or a small group of muscles. It occurs in persons of all ages, from infancy to old age. The muscle spasm is so violent that it brings the sleeper back to full wakefulness, in fact he is so aroused that it is often harder for him to get to sleep again than it was in the first place. The cause of these starts has never been determined, though they seem to be due to some temporary nervous tension. Thoroughgoing investigation by physiologists has established the fact that they have their origin in the cerebrum, the thinking part of the brain. Dr. Jacobson indicates that they occur even when sleep has been induced by his methods of relaxation. *It is however a striking fact that when sleep is induced by controlled breathing as outlined in this book, the sleep start becomes conspicuous by its absence. It almost never occurs.* The present writer cannot recall that he has ever experienced a sleep start after putting himself to sleep by this procedure, though at other times he has his share of this trouble. The truth is that he often uses the breathing procedures when he would not need them as far as sleep is concerned, but just as an insurance that he will not be awakened by a sleep start. The prevention of these starts, which could hardly have been predicted beforehand, would seem to indicate that the carbon dioxide accumulated by controlled breathing is highly effective in securing relaxation, and that this is accomplished by quieting the nervous system, including the highest centers of the brain.

Summary: Put on the Brakes to Slow Down for Sleep

To sum up the discussion of relaxation, bear in mind: (1). The person who is living under entirely normal conditions does not need to read a book or to go through a course of training in order to learn how to relax sufficiently to meet nature's requirement for going to sleep. He only needs to lie down in a comfortable, quiet place, and nature does the rest. He does not even need to control his breathing beyond the automatic control that nature gives him.

(2). Living as we do, however, under the highly artificial conditions of the present, where muscular fatigue is at a minimum and nervous tension is high, many of us find our reactions somewhat abnormal. At the end of the day we have an accumulated activity momentum which does not come to an automatic stop, and this calls for aid of some kind, some sort of braking action, to slow down our activity momentum enough to make sleep possible.

In this situation the important consideration is that this braking action should be secured by some method that is natural and wholesome rather than artificial and harmful, and that the means used should be easily accessible, not inconvenient, not laborious or unpleasant, and yet effective in bringing the necessary slowing down into sleep. These requirements, it is believed, are fully met by the procedures which are described in this book. In the first place, they secure relaxation by means of the body's own natural relaxer, carbon dioxide, which calms both nerves and muscles in all parts of the body, including also the brain, without conscious attention except to breathing. (3). These procedures cause no inconvenience, need no previous planning, require no serious effort. And best of all, they are entirely wholesome, completely harmless, and absolutely safe.

12. Muscle fatigue, mental fatigue, and nervous fatigue

Do They All Help Us Sleep?

The popular conception of the relation of fatigue to sleep is expressed in the saying, "I'm tired enough to sleep without rocking," meaning that if one is sufficiently tired nothing else is required to ensure sleep. As applied to ordinary muscular fatigue, and within certain limits, the idea embodied in this saying is correct. But different kinds of fatigue, as we shall see, may have very different effects.

Fatigue resulting from muscular activity manifests itself in three ways. First, in a reduction of the capacity to perform work; second, in chemical changes in the muscles; and third, in a subjective feeling of tiredness which may be described as a disinclination to put forth effort. The first of these effects, the reduction of work output, may indicate the presence of conditions which would affect sleep, but in itself it has nothing to do with sleep. The second effect, chemical change in the muscles, is principally an accumulation of lactic acid which occurs during severe muscular exertion. This condition is so quickly cleared away when exertion stops and ample oxygen is again available that it does not extend into the time when one would expect to sleep. The third effect, the feeling of tiredness and disinclination to effort, is the one which is significant for sleep. This feeling commonly results from moderate muscular exercise which has been continued for a considerable length of time.

The physiological cause of this feeling of tiredness is not definitely known. It may be connected with the deterioration of the Nissl granules of the nerve cells which accompanies fatigue, or with other changes in the nerves, or it may be related to changes in hormone secretion. No significant changes in general bodily conditions have been found to accompany ordinary muscular fatigue. Careful measurements at the Harvard fatigue laboratory failed to detect any changes even after a hard day's work, though when judged by his feelings the worker was quite tired. The sleep-producing effect of this feeling is undoubtedly due in part at least to the muscular relaxation which accompanies it. When we feel a strong aversion to muscular exertion our brains stop sending out contraction impulses to our muscles, and the muscles relax. Relaxed muscles send a greatly reduced number of activity reports to the brain. Authorities on sleep agree that reduction of these muscle reports is a necessary condition of sleep and an important, if not the major, factor in producing it.

While moderate muscular exercise can produce relaxation, which is an aid to sleep, muscular exercise carried to extremes can produce conditions which are a serious hindrance to sleep. Moderate muscular fatigue is not felt in the muscles. Its only manifestation is in the mind, subjective, a desire to avoid further exertion. But muscular exertion, even when moderate, if continued too long will bring muscular soreness which can make sleep difficult. Muscles not accustomed to exercise can develop soreness very quickly, due to the accumulation of lactic acid and other products of contraction. This type of soreness is usually felt within a short time after the exercise is stopped. It can be relieved by use of a liniment or heat to dilate the blood vessels combined with periods of light exercise or massage to stimulate the circulation and thus carry away the irritants that have accumulated. Soreness of this type can be prevented by suitable preparatory training of the muscles. Training increases the blood supply of the muscles and thus prevents the accumulation of waste products.

A different type of muscle soreness sometimes follows extreme muscular effort. It is due to actual physical damage to the muscle, such as tearing some of the muscle fibers. Muscles that are not often used are most susceptible to such injury. The resulting soreness or lameness is felt in a very definite location, but usually does not become painful until some hours after the injury occurs. As treatment, rest of the muscle is most important. Heat is beneficial, and liniment may reduce soreness. Occasional light use of the muscle helps to avoid adhesions between the injured muscle fibers.

While we usually think of fatigue in connection with our muscles, the term is often applied to conditions which have little or no connection with the muscles. One such condition is often called mental fatigue. Whether the mind itself is subject to fatigue is extremely doubtful. Careful tests indicate that problems in mental arithmetic can be solved as rapidly and as accurately after a long period of work at similar tasks as when there had been no previous period of such work. It seems likely that the condition commonly called mental fatigue is a sort of boredom brought about by the conditions under which the work is done. Heat and humidity, also holding the body in one position, or just working in unpleasant company, can bring on the feeling of tiredness.

The most probable mental cause that can be suggested for this mental fatigue is the effort required to keep the attention fixed on the task. This effort varies inversely with the degree of interest the worker has in the work. Mental work in which one is intensely interested causes little or no fatigue. Mental fatigue, so called, usually manifests itself as boredom, relaxation, and eventually as sleepiness. No doubt mental fatigue would aid sleep if it could be induced at an appropriate time. It can usually be relieved by moderate physical exercise.

Nervous or Chronic Fatigue Makes Us Jumpy

A condition very different from either muscular or mental

fatigue has been called nervous fatigue. It is characterized by irritability and jumpiness, the nervous system responding in an exaggerated manner to any kind of stimulus. This is a condition very important in any consideration of sleep, because it makes sleep almost impossible until it can be relieved. It is the principal cause of the present widespread use of sleeping pills, which of course can give only temporary relief and are likely to produce even worse trouble.

Nervous fatigue has also been called chronic fatigue, because of its persistence. It is most often caused by working over a period of time under strong pressure of some kind, such as hurry to meet a certain deadline, anxiety as to the possible outcome of an undertaking, or worry from any one of many possible causes, also by habitually continuing to work beyond the point of normal fatigue or by failing to get sufficient sleep. Nervous fatigue does not lead to rest and recovery as muscular fatigue does. The anxiety and worry which caused it, by preventing rest, continue to aggravate the condition until they are relieved.

Nervous fatigue might very well be called emotional fatigue, because the emotions are directly concerned both in its origin and in its effects. But physical conditions are also involved, both as cause and as effect. In seeking a cure, predisposing causes as well as immediate causes must be sought in both fields, and relief sought in either or both as the individual case may require.

When we consider the conditions of modern life it is not surprising that nervous fatigue is so prevalent. The radio, telephone, automobile, and airplane have speeded up the tempo of life far beyond the pace for which our bodies, especially our nervous systems, were designed. The impacts to which our senses and our higher nervous centers must respond have been multiplied beyond anything that was imaginable a hundred years ago. Worse still, the nature of the problems which we must face have undergone radical changes. Instead of simple and tangible difficulties which could be easily discerned and directly attacked, we are now confronted by complicated and abstract problems which are difficult to understand and offer no direct line of attack. In grappling with such problems we necessarily meet with failure more often than with success. Unless we can find in life something that is deeply satisfying and largely independent of our temporary successes or failures, the strain of the multiplied frustrations is quite likely to lead to the condition which we have called nervous fatigue.

Nervous fatigue can be recognized by the fact that it bears no relation to work done or exertion put forth, and that it is not relieved by rest or even by such sleep as can be obtained. It is usually worse in the morning and more or less relieved toward evening, with physical exertion tending to increase the relief. Nervous fatigue is always a decidedly disagreeable sensation as contrasted with ordinary muscular fatigue, which normally is a rather pleasant feeling.

In the treatment of nervous fatigue the first essential is to make sure that there is no serious physical disease or deficiency which could account for it. However, its source is much more likely to be found in the circumstances and conditions under which the patient lives and works. Here careful scrutiny will probably discover the emotional stresses which are responsible, though physical factors in the surroundings may be involved and must not be overlooked. Removal of unfavorable conditions will usually be followed by rapid recovery. But nervous fatigue when allowed to continue over long periods may cause unwholesome physical or even mental conditions, and such conditions may call for specific treatment to ensure recovery.

Tired Businessman and His Hunger Fatigue.   A type of nervous fatigue which is becoming too frequent among business and professional men might be called in plain language hunger fatigue. A physiologist or doctor would be most likely to call it hypoglycemic fatigue, referring to the reduced quantity of sugar (glucose) in the blood. This type of fatigue has been extensively discussed by Doctor Sidney A. Portis and his associates at Michael Reese Hospital, Chicago, in the Journal of the American Medical Association, a very comprehensive discussion appearing in the issue for

Dec. 2, 1950, under the title, "Exhaustion in the Young Business Executive." In many cases, probably in most, this type of fatigue, though its immediate cause could be classed as hunger, is not felt as hunger at all, but as increased difficulty or exasperation with the work which the person is trying to do, or as discomfort resulting from the conditions under which he is working, or even as annoyance with the shortcomings, real or imaginary, of his assistants. He becomes irritable and impatient and finds it difficult to concentrate.

Because most of the energy of the body and all the energy of the brain comes from the oxidation (burning) of glucose, an adequate and continuous supply of this sugar in the blood is necessary for everyone, whether his job is day labor or the highest type of brain work. Glucose is often injected into the veins of a sick person who cannot secure nourishment through his stomach, for this kind of sugar can be used in the body as it is without going through the process of digestion. Ordinarily it is made in the body by various body chemicals acting on the foods which we eat. A certain amount of it in a concentrated form called glycogen is stored in the body, principally in the liver and the muscles. These stores are drawn upon between meals when the digestion of foods has been completed and glucose is no longer coming into the blood from the food. In the physically inactive businessman these stores may not become available until after the blood sugar level has fallen below normal. The result is that in the interval before the stores of glycogen have become available there is a reduction of the brain's energy supply which brings on hunger fatigue.

Ordinary sugar (sucrose), because it requires very little change during digestion, can supply glucose to the blood more quickly than most other kinds of food. The starch foods, such as bread and cereals, require more change and are a little longer in reaching the blood than the sugars. The various fats, including butter and cream, take longer than the starches to become available for the body's use, while the protein foods, such as lean meat, fish, eggs, cheese, milk, and nuts, require still longer, and so, as we commonly say, they "stick to the ribs" for a longer time. This difference in the time required for digestion of the three principal types of food is one of the strongest arguments for eating balanced meals. Such meals supply glucose to the blood at a more even rate and for a longer time.

Dr. Portis examined a large group of business executives who complained of the symptoms of nervous fatigue. He found that when their blood sugar level was raised by injections of glucose it would fall again very quickly, losing all the increase within an hour, and then continuing to fall during another two hours, in the end being much below a normal amount. Something caused the glucose to disappear from their blood too quickly and too completely. Consequently when they ate the average businessman's hurried breakfast of coffee and toast or cereal, heavily sweetened, the resulting quick increase of blood sugar no doubt followed the same course as the glucose injection. It was disposed of quickly, with a period of low blood sugar following. If lunch was light and principally of carbohydrate foods, sugars and starches, it could give only temporary relief to be followed by another period of low blood sugar. The brain, getting its energy entirely from glucose, is especially sensitive to this deficiency, and the result is hunger fatigue. *In this condition smoking will give some relief, but unfortunately it does this not by supplying more glucose but by increasing the use of the already limited supply, so that the final result is a worsening of the condition with often a resort to chain smoking.*

This abnormally rapid and extended reduction of blood glucose following a carbohydrate meal traces back to the over-activity of the pancreatic gland. This is the gland which produces insulin, a hormone that enables the body to oxidize glucose for the production of heat and energy. If this gland fails it causes diabetes, which can only be relieved by injections of insulin obtained from animals. While a proper supply of insulin is necessary to life, too much of it causes low blood sugar and hinders all activities of the body, but especially those of the brain, where its first effect is a feeling of uneasiness and irritation.

Two causes contribute to the over-secretion of insulin with its resultant low blood sugar. In the first place, a meal that consists largely of sugar and starch floods the blood with glucose and stimulates the secretion of insulin to dispose of the temporary over-supply. With the repetition of such meals this over-secretion becomes habitual. As a second cause, the pancreatic gland is subject to nervous stimulation, and nervous tension of any kind tends to increase its secretion. So when the business executive, after his starch and sugar breakfast, meets even the normal tensions of his business day, this nervous strain is added to the habitual over-secretion of his pancreatic gland, and rapid exhaustion of his blood sugar with its accompanying irritability and fatigue necessarily follows.

Most of the glucose which disappears so rapidly from the blood when there is an over-secretion of insulin seems to be changed largely to fat and stored in the body's various fat depots. Apparently when the sugar has been stored as fat an interval of time is required to recall it for the body's use. This would account for the period of low blood sugar which follows an over-supply of glucose. It may account also for a tendency to accumulate fat with resulting over-weight, for when the discovery is once made that the unpleasantness of low blood sugar can be relieved by eating (or drinking) sugar, this will usually be resorted to before the fat reserves can be mobilized. So most of the stored fat accumulates in the reserves, increasing the waistline and the weight.

Correcting Hunger Fatigue

To correct this hunger fatigue, if the condition has not continued too long, improvement of the diet together with a determination to take it easy at the office may be all that is required. A glass of milk may be taken in the forenoon if desired, also another in the afternoon. This will help to tide over any temporary fall of the blood sugar level. At all meals a strict limitation of sweets, with a fair amount of starches, some fat, and liberal quantities of protein should be the rule. In long continued or more stubborn cases a physician can prescribe drugs to limit the nervous stimulation of the pancreatic gland and to reduce its over-activity. All sources of nervous tension, whether in business or outside, should be reduced as far as possible. Some pleasant and absorbing, but not too strenuous, activity should be arranged for leisure hours. In extremely difficult cases it may be necessary to consult a competent psychiatrist.

And now what does this long discussion of hunger fatigue have to do with sleep? Simply this: Hunger fatigue with its jitteriness and nervous excitability is by no means limited to business hours. It can and does occur also during the hours that should be devoted to sleep. And it is even a greater hindrance to restful sleep than it is to business efficiency. Though the tensions of the business day may be absent, habitual over-activity of insulin secretion may exhaust the blood sugar from the evening meal before bedtime. This is especially apt to occur if considerable time or any strenuous activity comes between. And when the business executive takes his business worries to bed with him he faces the same combined effect of habitual over-activity and nervous stimulation of his pancreatic gland that he would be subject to at his office. The frequent occurrence of this condition of low blood sugar at night is the reason why so many writers on sleep recommend a light snack before bedtime.

Under conditions of hunger fatigue sleep usually comes only with complete exhaustion, and not really restful sleep at that, for with the blood sugar below normal, energy is not available for the restorative processes that should go on during sleep. And the brain is the greatest sufferer from poor sleep. As the late Dr. George Crile pointed out long ago, it seems to be the brain rather than other parts of the body which requires sleep for its recuperation. Recent studies have shown that while most other parts of the body have greatly reduced activity and energy consumption during sleep, the brain requires, as far as can be determined, just as much glucose

and oxygen for its activities during sleep as during vigorous thinking in the waking hours. For a clear and vigorous brain when
awake, fully recuperative sleep is absolutely essential.

When there is reason to believe that low blood sugar is the cause
of restlessness at night or of too long a period of wakefulness
before going to sleep, a glass of milk with a few crackers or some
cereal before retiring should be tried. The first effect of low blood
sugar on the brain is not to dull or quiet it but rather to irritate
it and make it more excitable, causing what we sometimes call
jitteriness or jumpiness. In this condition the bedtime snack can
make sleep possible when without it getting to sleep in a reasonable
time would be difficult or impossible.

Sleep difficulty from low blood sugar, or hunger fatigue, does not
always come at the time of retiring. Sometimes it is not felt until
after an hour or two of sleep, when it causes wakefulness and
difficulty in getting to sleep again. When this occurs it is best to
get up, sip a glass of milk and munch a few crackers while reading
something interesting but not exciting. On returning to bed sleep
will often come quickly, or will yield promptly to use of the
breathing exercises.

Under normal conditions of rest while awake the body's stores
of glycogen in the liver are sufficient to maintain an adequate
blood sugar level for several hours. During sleep less energy is
required than when resting while awake. So when all body functions are normal the glycogen store should be sufficient to go
through the night without the need of supplementing the supply
by eating. But when through poor food habits or unusual nervous
tension the normal processes of the body are disturbed, or when
in older persons the glycogen supply from the liver may not become available promptly, there is apt to be a disturbing period of
low blood sugar. When this condition occurs it should not be met
with drugs like alcohol or tobacco, or by the brain-paralyzing
effects of sleeping pills. It is far better to supplement the falling
blood sugar with a light snack to bridge the gap. Once the liver
glycogen is mobilized it is likely to carry through the night without

further disturbance. Of course, in stubborn cases, this night-time hunger fatigue may, like the daytime phase, require remedial treatment by a physician.

Summary: Eat Right, Adjust and Sleep

Of the three types of fatigue, muscular, mental, and nervous, nervous fatigue is by far the greatest obstacle to sleep. Hunger fatigue is, of course, only one type of nervous fatigue, and as indicated above, it will usually yield to simple and direct measures, primarily a well-chosen diet.

Other types of nervous fatigue are frequently due to maladjustment in one's pattern of living and to excessive emotional conflicts and strains. When such conditions are of a merely temporary and passing nature the primary need is to secure sleep until the conditions improve, and the procedures described in this book are ideally suited for this purpose. Whenever nervous fatigue does not yield to these procedures it may be necessary to seek psychiatric treatment before natural sleep can be secured.

Chronic tiredness may sometimes be caused by insufficiency of the thyroid hormone due to lack of iodine in the body. If suitable tests show insufficiency of this hormone, it should be prescribed in pill form. In rare cases symptoms similar to those of nervous or chronic fatigue may accompany the beginning of disease of the nerves, such as muscular dystrophy or *myasthenia gravis,* requiring the attention of a specialist.

13. How to make your eyes
put you to sleep

Our Two Daily Acts

When we intend to go to sleep we always do two things. We lie down and we close our eyes. These two acts, though they may seem very different, both serve a common purpose. Each act interrupts a flood of nerve impulses being constantly sent to the brain during our normal waking activities. Such nerve impulses stimulate the thinking part of our brains into alertness, and under ordinary conditions prevent the approach of sleep. When we are engaged in any kind of activity, or even just holding our bodies in a standing or sitting position, the muscles used are constantly sending reports of their activities to the brain. When we lie down these muscles go out of use and stop sending their reports. This is what we call relaxation. Here we will consider what part the eyes can play in bringing sleep through the limitation of their reports to the brain.

Two quite different groups of nerve impulses come to the brain from the eyes. One group carries the visual images which are produced by the rays of light focused upon the retina at the back of the eyeball by the lens of the eye. This group of impulses is cut off almost completely when the eyes are closed. But the eyelids are not actually opaque. They are slightly translucent, so that in bright light scattered rays pass through them. This light cannot be focused by the lens to produce images on the retina, but it does keep the retina alerted and the brain aware of the presence of light. It is because of this that bedrooms should be dark or at most only dimly lighted. If it is necessary to sleep in bright light, the eyelids should be covered with a pair of comfortable eye shades. Under ordinary conditions this group of nerve impulses is easy to control.

The second group of nerve impulses from the eyes is much less easily controlled, and very few writers on sleep have attacked the problem. This group comes from the muscles that move the eyeballs, keeping the eyes pointed accurately toward the things we wish to see. They, like all muscles, constantly send reports of their activities to the brain. It might be supposed that when the eyelids are closed and the eyes are not being used for seeing these muscles would necessarily be inactive, and therefore would have no messages to send to the brain. That this is not the case can be quickly appreciated by closing the eyes and then noting what happens when the thoughts are turned from one side of the room to the other. Movements of the eyeballs quite distinctly follow the thoughts. Evidently closing the eyelids does not stop the activity of the muscles that move the eyeballs. Conscious efforts to control them are useless. They are under the unconscious control of the thoughts, and the only way to control them is by the indirect method of controlling the thoughts.

There are several reasons why control of these eyeball muscles is important in bringing sleep. They are the most delicate and finely organized muscles in the body, quite different in their make-up from other muscles. They are supplied with a large number of highly sensitive nerve endings, called muscle spindles, which send messages from the muscles to the brain. The area of the brain devoted to control of these muscles is far greater in proportion to their size than is usual for other muscles of the body. These muscles use oxygen at a much higher rate for their size than any other muscles, indicating that they are capable of much more intense activity than other muscles. The nerves from the eye muscles connect with a center in the brain which is very close to the sleep control center, and it seems probable that the activities of the two centers are closely associated.

The important bearing of these muscles upon sleep is demonstrated in a practical way by the number of popular sleep rituals which depend upon or at least include some special use of the eyes. There are many variations, but all tend to fatigue the eye muscles, or in some way to reduce their activity. Usually the inventors and proponents of these rituals are completely unaware that the success of the rituals in bringing sleep is due in any way to these muscles or to their control. Fortunately ignorance of how the ritual works does not prevent it from working, and it is true that in many cases, if wakefulness did not yield to the ordinary preparations for sleep, a slight control of this group of muscles might be all that was required to tip the balance and bring sleep.

What Happens When You Turn Your Eyes Upward

Many years ago a book was published in Cleveland, Ohio, under the peculiar title, *Knowledge Enhanced*. Its author, Luther Stockton Fish, was an acute observer of objective facts, and he was an ingenious inventor of plausible theories to account for the observed facts. He had observed in a large number of cases that persons who turned their eyes strongly upward and persistently held them in that position for a considerable time almost invariably became drowsy, and in not a few cases actually went to sleep, even though they were not in bed and had not planned to sleep. Trying out the idea, he found that he was often able to put himself to sleep this way.

Having convinced himself that there was a definite connection between this upward position of the eyes and the coming of sleep, he began searching for an explanation. Knowing that there was evidence of electrical activity in the brain, and using his limited knowledge of the brain's anatomy, he proceeded to build a theory. He started with the assumption that thought is dependent on the flow of an electrical current in the brain, and that the flow of this current is dependent on immediate contact, as it is in a metallic circuit. As the site of a make-and-break contact he chose the mamillary bodies, since they are so placed that they might easily be in contact or separated. The mamillary bodies are two nodular groups of brain cells in the central, lower, back part of the brain. When these mamillary bodies were in contact, according to his theory, electrical current could flow between the two sides of the brain. This, he thought, would make thinking possible, and the person would be awake. When this contact was broken thought would be impossible, and the result would be sleep. He accounted for the making and breaking of the mamillary contact by attributing it to the position of the eyes. When the eyes were turned down, as they usually are in ordinary activities, they would, he thought, exert a pull on the optic nerve, and this would draw the mamillary bodies into contact. When the eyes turned upward this pull would no longer be exerted and the contact would be broken, bringing sleep.

Mr. Fish's theory of sleep, like too many others, depended on assumptions for its validity, and it was not valid because his assumptions were in conflict with hard facts. To cite only one of these facts, the optic nerve is firmly anchored to the skull where it emerges into the eye socket, and it is provided with ample slack outside to take up eye movements, so that it cannot possibly exert a pull on any part of the brain.

A false theory to account for observed facts does not however, in any way invalidate the facts. When I discovered Mr. Fish's book in the library of Wittenberg College I recognized at once that his theory was impossible, but I also realized that his observations both confirmed and explained my own observation that watching rockets exploding or my spirit floating away above me was much more effective in bringing sleep than counting sheep was. It was clearly the position of my eyes that had made the difference.

Proofs from Sleeping Soldiers

Discarding the false theory which Mr. Fish had advanced did not automatically give me a better one to take its place. And much searching through books and scientific journals dealing with the eye brought very little light on the subject. The first clue to authoritative confirmation and a more acceptable explanation came when Dale Carnegie published his book, *How to Stop Worrying and Start Living*. In it he mentions briefly that Dr. Foster Kennedy had used this method in putting himself to sleep. Tracing this clue, I later found Dr. Kennedy's own account of his discovery of the merits of this procedure, which he had published in the New York State Journal of Medicine. Dr. Kennedy was a prominent neurologist of New York City, professor of neurology at Cornell Medical College, and neurological chief at Belleview Hospital. So his discovery, use and recommendation of this method of bringing sleep seemed to be about as high a certification of its validity as I could hope to find. Dr. Kennedy wrote that during World War I he examined the eyes of soldiers who had fallen asleep in utter exhaustion, and that their eyes were always turned strongly upward. Taking a suggestion from this he began experimenting on himself, purposely putting his eyes in a similar position, and in a short time he began to feel sleepy. As a result he adopted this device as a regular method of wooing sleep. He described it as "an automatic associated reflex over which I had no voluntary control."

The late Sir Charles Sherrington, a Nobel prize winner, demonstrated that all parts of the human body, including the brain, are linked together in an infinitely complex system of what are called reflex arcs. These arcs consist of a nerve which brings in a sensation, one or more central relay points, and a nerve which carries the action response out to a muscle or gland. Nearly all of our life processes are maintained by these reflex arcs, many of them conditioned, the others innate. In most cases no awareness of these reflexes ever reaches the conscious mind, and when it does it is only after the response has already occurred.

The eyelids of a baby close instantly whenever it sees a hand or other object coming too close. This is what we call an instinctive action or an inborn reflex. The baby does not need to learn it by being hit in the eye. But the baby does not know that he should keep his hand away from a hot stove until after he has been burned. Once burned he withdraws his hands quickly at the first sensation of heat, and soon this action becomes quicker than thought, like an inborn reflex. This learned automatic response to the sensation of heat is what physiologists call a conditioned reflex. At first our salivary glands secrete saliva only when we taste or smell food. But soon they get the habit of secreting saliva when we see the food, or even at the sound of the dinner bell if we are very hungry, though we have as yet neither tasted nor smelled the food. This response of the salivary glands to sight or sound is a learned, or conditioned, reflex.

It seems likely that what Dr. Kennedy meant to tell us is that since the upward position of the eyeballs is the position of rest which they regularly take as we fall asleep, we have learned to associate it so closely with sleep that it can bring about the involuntary act of falling asleep, just as the sight of food can bring about the involuntary act of secreting saliva. We cannot will either going to sleep or the secretion of saliva, but both can be brought about by other acts over which we do have voluntary control. We only need to learn what these other acts are, and to use them.

In a sense all our habitual preparations for sleep tend to become the starting point of what may be called reflex action leading to sleep. These preparations, being often repeated, become firmly fixed as part of the process of going to sleep. But turning of the eyes upward seems to exert a more powerful effect in bringing sleep than could be expected from habit alone. Part of this effect is no doubt due to the concentration of attention which is necessary to keep the eyes in this position, because this prevents the mind from wandering to disturbing thoughts. In addition voluntary effort probably pulls the eyes up beyond their normal resting position, and this quickly brings in another strong aid to sleep, fatigue of the eye muscles.

Both Dr. Kennedy and Mr. Fish agree that the turning of the eyes upward is not always sufficient to bring sleep when used alone, and both suggest ways of adding to the effects of the eye position. Dr. Kennedy emphasizes voluntary relaxation of the body muscles. Mr. Fish proposes the forming of mental pictures as a means of controlling the thoughts, a procedure which is fully discussed in Appendix A in connection with the supplemental type of breathing. Neither of them considers the part that may be played by the effort of keeping the eyes up, either in fatigue of the eye muscles or in holding the attention.

An article by J. E. Lebanson appeared in the Archives of Ophthalmology for March, 1941, under almost the same title as this chapter, "The Eye and Sleep." It is a real storehouse of information regarding various relations between the eyes and sleep, but it does not take up the question of how the eyes can aid in bringing sleep. The article calls attention to the fact that after long wakefulness the eyes show many signs of fatigue, indicating how necessary it is for them to have the rest that only sleep can bring. It also brings out the interesting points that the closing of the eyelids in sleep is an instinctive act, being present in newborn babies, while the turning of the eyes upward is an acquired habit, being present in only a small per cent of babies and very young children. This upward position of the eyes is called the resting position, which implies of course that in this position the eye muscles can be expected to be less active, with fewer impulses sent to the brain, though no suggestion is made of a possible connection between this resting position and the coming of sleep.

Summary: A Multiple Combination of Natural Aids

The procedures proposed in this book are planned to take the fullest possible advantage of the help that the eyes can give in bringing sleep, including Dr. Kennedy's automatic reflex and Mr. Fish's mental picture forming, as well as eye muscle fatigue and attention-holding effort. Relaxation of both eye and body muscles is also included, but principally on an unconscious and involuntary basis rather than by direct effort.

The main purpose of all our procedures is to increase the blood's content of carbon dioxide with its specific and positive quieting effects on the nerves and the brain and its relaxation of the muscles. (See Chapter 16.)

With this multiple combination of natural aids to sleep available, there can be little justification for a person in ordinary health resorting to the use of sleep-producing drugs with their stupefying effects and their risk of leading to a life-wrecking drug habit.

14. Are cat naps worthwhile?

How Churchill Benefited

Probably there is no better way to begin this chapter than by quoting the following passage from Sir Winston Churchill:

"I have had recourse to a method of life which greatly extended my daily capacity for work.

"I always went to bed at least for one hour as early as possible in the afternoon and exploited to the full my happy gift of falling almost immediately into deep sleep. By this means I was able to press a day and a half's work into one.

"Nature had not intended mankind to work from eight in the morning until midnight without that refreshment of blessed oblivion, which, even if it only lasts twenty minutes, is sufficient to renew all the vital forces.

"I regretted having to send myself to bed like a child every afternoon, but I was rewarded by being able to work through the night until two or even later—sometimes much later—in the morning, and begin the new day between eight and nine o'clock. This routine I observed throughout the war, and I commend it to others if and when they find it necessary for a long spell to get the last scrap out of the human structure."

In this passage Sir Winston recognizes the inconvenience, or even humiliation, of his addiction to the afternoon nap, but he indicates that these objections are far outweighed, in his opinion, by the great increase in work output which it makes possible. He hints that there is a physiological basis for this increase of output by saying that nature had not intended mankind to work long hours without sleep. It is to be noted further that he does not recommend his practice as desirable for everyone, but only for those who "find it necessary for a long spell to get the last scrap out of the human machine."

The three points Sir Winston makes as to the inconvenience, the increased efficiency, and the physiological basis of the afternoon nap will be considered in this chapter, because these points should all be weighed carefully by anyone who considers adopting such a plan. Unfortunately the napping habit is not one that lends itself to temporary or intermittent use. Though it may prove a permanent gain, once adopted it is likely to be also a permanent handicap in our society, which is geared to a single period of sleep at night.

How the Author Benefited

When the present writer was paying his way through college by working during the summer vacations as a specialty salesman he discovered by chance the difference that a mid-day nap can make in a person's effectiveness during the afternoon and evening. The business of a specialty salesman does not go forward by its own momentum. It moves only as the salesman pushes it. His sales register at once any increase or decrease in his effectiveness.

After lunch one day I was so overcome by fatigue that I decided to lie down for a few minutes' rest. I awoke nearly an hour later worried because of the time lost—wasted as I then considered it. Interviewing prospective customers, however, I soon noticed how much more alert I was than usual. This alertness continued through the afternoon and evening and resulted in sales greater than I had made in any day previously. Profiting by this experience I made the after-lunch nap a standard part of my sales promotion program.

On returning to college I tested the midday nap on my studies and found that by sleeping half-an-hour after lunch I could continue studying for an hour longer at night. Also I was more clear-headed and retained more of the subjects I covered. It seemed foolish to throw away this increased accomplishment, so I continued the midday nap through both college and university.

After leaving school it happened that my work permitted me to continue the midday naps. During periods when I had only an hour off at noon I still managed to get fifteen or twenty minutes of sleep. Now, close to ninety, and no longer on a fixed schedule I sleep about an hour after lunch. I think these naps are largely responsible for my present degree of health and continued mental alertness.

Avoid Accumulating Fatigue

Apparently the physiological principle which largely accounts for the benefits of midday sleep is the accelerated rate at which fatigue accumulates when work is continued without break. Many years ago Frank Gilbreth, a pioneer in industrial efficiency, clearly realized this characteristic of fatigue. He and his wife Lillian, parents of the family made famous by the book, *Cheaper by the Dozen,* in their book, *Fatigue Study,* put the matter plainly as follows: "We know that exertion not only uses up temporarily the energy of the body, but that it also seems to generate a sort of poison which 'slows one down' for the time being . . . we know also that the effects of fatigue are more difficult to overcome as the fatigue becomes greater. Careful observation and records show that a little fatigue is easily overcome if proper rest is supplied immediately. Twice the amount of fatigue requires more than twice the amount of rest. Four times the amount of fatigue demands more than twice as much rest as the preceding 'more than twice the amount of rest,' until, finally, a state of excessive fatigue requires a rest period that might have to be prolonged indefinitely."

If we wish to reduce the matter to figures, we might say that if we assign a value of 100 units to the fatigue caused by two hours of exertion, then the number of units of fatigue produced by a second two hours of continuous exertion is greater than 100, let us say 125, so that the total fatigue units for the four hours is not 200 but 225. Continuing these illustrative figures, the third two hours might rate 175, and a fourth two hours probably 300. Thus the total for an eight-hour day would not be four times the fatigue units for the first two hours, that is, 400, but instead would be 700, which is nearly double what it would have been if the rate of fatigue production had remained the same as in the first two hours. Probably the figures used here would be applicable only to very heavy work. But the principle applies to all continuous exertion, though the rate of fatigue acceleration will of course vary as exertion becomes more or less severe.

After eight hours of continuous exertion most of us need eight hours of sleep for complete recuperation. But if we break this acceleration of fatigue by stopping at the end of each two hours for a period of sleep we can make a fresh start, and thus produce only 100 units of fatigue for each two hours of exertion. And because we have the lower total of fatigue to recover from we do not require such a long period of sleep for recovery. Four periods of an hour or an hour-and-a-half of sleep, taken following each two-hour period of exertion will probably be sufficient. Thus four to six hours of sleep at intervals will give the same degree of recuperation as eight hours of sleep taken at the end of eight hours of continuous exertion.

The principle involved here is well illustrated by the operation of a water-power sawmill in southwest Virginia to which my father sometimes hauled sawlogs when I was a boy. The stream flow at the sawmill was considerably less most of the time than the amount of water required to operate the saw, even when the dam was full, giving maximum water pressure. Consequently when the mill was started and sawing began the height of water in the dam began to fall, and with this lowered pressure a greater volume of water had continually to be released through the turbine to maintain the power output. The second hour of sawing therefore required a considerably larger amount of water than had been used in the first hour. When there was an average stream flow, if sawing was stopped at the end of the first hour the dam would refill in half-an-hour and the mill was ready for a fresh start, using no more water in the second hour than it had in the first. But if the mill ran continuously for two hours at the start, the time required for refilling the dam was about an hour-and-a-half, because the lower pressure during the second hour made it necessary to use about twice as much water as in the first hour. This meant that the time required for refilling would now be three-fourths of the operating time, as against half of the operating time, as it was at the end of the first hour. During a third hour of continuous operation the water pressure ran down so rapidly and so much more water was used that four hours were necessary for refilling. This was a third more than the operating time, as compared with half the operating time when the mill was operated in one-hour periods. Any effort to operate the mill longer than three hours continuously on the usual stream flow was a waste of both time and water, for very soon the water pressure became so low that it would no longer operate the saw at all.

It is the acceleration of fatigue, so well illustrated by the old sawmill, that accounts for the frequently heard statement that an hour of sleep before midnight is worth two hours after midnight. The difference is not in the sleep, but in the fatigue. Extending the day's activities into those last hours before midnight brings a more rapid accumulation of fatigue, requiring more than a proportional lengthening of sleep for recuperation. Yet in practice it is apt to mean an actual shortening of the hours of sleep, since in order to meet the day's regular schedule one probably must wake at the same time he had been accustomed to wake when he retired earlier.

That an accelerating rate of fatigue in continuous exertion holds true in actual experience, and that short intervening periods of rest can overcome it, has been proved many times. An extreme example is found in Buckminster Fuller's "Dymaxion" sleep, this peculiar term being his own coinage from the words dynamic and maximum. This well-known and highly original architect and inventor chose a time for his experiment when his work would not be interrupted and when he could leave his drawing board and return to it at will. He found that by sleeping an average of half an hour out of each three-hour period, day and night, he could keep fresh and alert during twenty hours of each day. After several months on this schedule a medical check-up showed him to be in prime condition.

Great Men Who Napped Often

Most of the commonly circulated stories about men who could work efficiently on much less sleep than the customary eight hours a day can be traced to this higher rate of recuperation in frequent short naps. Edison is often cited as an example of a long and highly creative life with very little sleep. It is true that when he was absorbed in an intensive investigation Edison sometimes went for long periods with much less than the standard eight hours of sleep, but it is now well established that he did it by interspersing naps in his laboratory between short periods of work. The couch in the library on which he slept can still be seen by visitors. Dr. Josephine Rathbone of Columbia University in her book *Teach Yourself to Relax,* reports a visit which her father, a newspaper man, made to Edison's laboratory. He found Edison sound asleep on a couch in the laboratory, and had to wake him for the interview. Edison explained that it was his custom to sleep whenever his mind became wearied, and said that he did not often work longer than four hours between naps. Alternating in this way his sleep was highly efficient, and probably was more extensive than the commonly reported four hours a day.

Another man, William Rainey Harper, first president of the University of Chicago, is often mentioned as a man who slept only four hours a day, and in his case the story is true and well verified. His case is exceptional in that he was able to work efficiently and to show prodigious accomplishments with only one period of four hours of sleep each night. Most people show such symptoms as irritability, foggy thinking, and depression after only a few nights with one short period of sleep. But when this same amount of sleep is broken up into several periods equally distributed through the twenty-four hours it will, for some people at least, maintain full efficiency.

In the case of Dr. Harper it is doubtful whether he gained in the end by his limited sleep, for he died at fifty with cancer of the stomach, an age when he should have been in his prime. It is quite possible that his short hours of sleep shortened his life and cost him more time than he gained. Napoleon Bonaparte is another man often mentioned as needing little sleep, but he, too, died at the age of fifty-two, and of the same disease, cancer of the stomach.

Harry Truman while president of the United States made it his rule to sleep about an hour after lunch. Also he made it his rule not to extend his waking day beyond eleven-thirty at night. During his successful campaign for reelection his stamina and endurance were a source of wonder and surprise to the whole country. Jonathan Daniels, who traveled in Mr. Truman's campaign party, thinks that his continued vigor and alertness were due to the fact that whenever there was a break of as much as thirty minutes in campaign activities he would lie down and take a nap. Since completing his seven years in the supposedly man-killing job of president, Mr. Truman is still strong and vigorous, and active in the affairs of his party. Our much-admired President Theodore (Teddy) Roosevelt followed a similar practice of napping on his campaign trips. It is well known that Ex-President Dwight Eisenhower, since his heart attack, is under strict orders from his doctors to take an hour's nap after lunch every day in the hope of warding off another heart attack. Former Senate Majority Leader, Lyndon B. Johnson, later Vice-President, was placed under similar orders as a result of a similar attack. Such orders, of course, raise the question whether an earlier adoption of this practice might not have prevented their first attacks.

The Best Time to Take a Daytime Nap

Whether to make a practice of taking an afternoon nap is a question every person must settle for himself, weighing against

E

its undoubted benefits the loss of time in the business day. Some persons take a nap at the end of the day's work, though this time is too late to yield the greatest benefit. Even a very short nap wedged in at the noon hour is better than waiting until the end of the day. A very short nap at noon and a longer one immediately after work may be a possible and desirable combination.

Dr. Nathaniel Kleitman's studies have shown that the average person, sleeping only at night, does not have his peak of efficiency immediately after waking. Instead, his efficiency rises more or less gradually during the morning and reaches a high point at some time during the day. Then it recedes more or less rapidly until it reaches a low point near his usual time for sleeping again. In view of this it would seem probable that when a person regularly takes a nap in the middle of the day he is able to develop two points of high efficiency during the day instead of one. So far as the present writer knows this has never been tested by scientific measurements, but practical experience seems to prove that a person can measurably increase his total time of high efficiency by breaking the day into two parts with a nap between.

It has been claimed by some that lying quietly with the eyes closed is almost or quite equal to sleep as a means of rest and recuperation. This is of course hard to measure with any degree of accuracy. There are, however, some very definite indications that these two types of rest are not by any means to be classed as the same thing. In sleep the pupils of the eyes are always contracted, the degree of contraction varying with the depth of sleep. When lying awake with the eyes closed just the opposite condition is found, there is a marked dilation of the pupils. The pupils of the eyes are controlled by the unconscious part of the brain, a part which does not report its actions to consciousness. Evidently to this part of the brain resting quietly with the eyes closed is a very different thing from being asleep. The muscles that hold one's head up are under both conscious and unconscious control, and respond freely to either. When one is asleep they respond to neither. The head drops from an erect position when sleep comes. So here again we find a sharp distinction between wakefulness and sleep. The electroencephalograph shows a similar difference in the electrical activity of the brain. When lying awake with the eyes closed the brain waves are markedly different from the waves in sleep. So we are not justified in assuming that the rest secured while lying awake is equal to the recuperation afforded by sleep, or even a satisfactory substitute for it.

Summary: Get Your Sleep Out

In taking an afternoon nap it is desirable that one should not be waked but should sleep until waking is voluntary. If no time is set for waking it will be found that the length of sleep will vary according to the body's need, thus compensating for any unusual exertion during the forenoon or inadequate sleep during the previous night. In this way fatigue is relieved promptly and not allowed to accumulate or "soak in" and produce effects which tend to become chronic and hard to overcome.

Sir Winston Churchill calls his ability to fall asleep quickly a happy gift, and such it is. But not everyone has this gift. The present writer had it most of his life, but lost it through illness. It was his successful effort to compensate for this loss that led to his writing this book.

For one who decides to become a daytime napper the method of inducing sleep by means of controlled breathing and other natural aids, as outlined in this book, will prove to be the greatest possible help. Its convenience, rapidity of action, and complete absence of hangover make it ideally adapted for this purpose.

15. How to stop snoring—
your own—another's

Cause and Cure

There is no evidence that snoring adds to or subtracts from the restfulness of sleep, though it is usually considered an evidence of sound sleep. Snoring is objectionable because of the disturbance it may cause to others sleeping within hearing, as well as the humiliation and resentment it may bring on the snorer.

The noise of snoring is produced by the vibration of the soft palate, the back part of the roof of the mouth. This vibration is most apt to occur when the mouth is open and air is inhaled or exhaled through both nose and mouth at the same time. From this it is evident that anything that leads to mouth breathing will produce a tendency to snoring.

There is general agreement that sleeping on the back tends to cause snoring. In this position as soon as the muscles relax after one falls asleep the weight of the lower jaw tends to pull the mouth open. With the mouth open there is nothing to prevent the double current of air which causes vibration of the soft palate.

Any obstruction of the nasal passages which does not allow the air to pass freely is apt to cause the sleeper to open his mouth in order to breathe more freely. In such a case there may still be sufficient air passing through the nose to give the double current and cause vibrations. Of course if the nasal passages are completely stopped, as in the case of a severe head cold, so that all breathing is through the mouth, there is little likelihood of snoring.

Various remedies have been proposed for snoring, and patents have been taken out on anti-snoring devices. One patent is on a shield to be worn between the teeth and lips and extending back into the cheeks. It is so designed that when the mouth falls open the flow of air through the mouth is still sufficiently obstructed to prevent vibration of the soft palate. Another patent is on a chin rest supported by head straps so designed as to hold the mouth shut without causing discomfort. Another device now on sale is a snore ball to be fastened to the back of the pajamas. It is a hollow rubber ball with a whistle attached so that when the sleeper turns on his back the air escaping from the ball will blow the whistle. The sound of the whistle is supposed to wake the sleeper and cause him to change his position. (It would seem that a tennis ball in a pocket on the back of the pajamas would be just as likely to wake the snorer, with less danger of waking his bed mate.)

See Your Doctor, Then Train Yourself

The first corrective action for the habitual snorer to take is to see a competent nose and throat specialist and make sure that his air passages are normal. The nasal passages may be obstructed by adenoids or a tumor, or a sinus discharge may cause obstruction. Sometimes the soft palate with its attached uvula is abnormally long. This will increase the vibration and make the snoring louder.

The snorer's second corrective action should be to train himself in the two habits of nose breathing and sleeping on his side. Avoidance of mouth breathing during his waking hours will help greatly in gaining the first of these habits. A comfortable pad the size of one's fist fitted under the chin when retiring and held in place by an elastic band around the neck will aid in extending the habit into the hours of sleep. Once this habit is fixed it will greatly reduce the tendency to snoring.

A snorer should make it a rule always to lie on his side when going to sleep. Often this can be extended into a habit of sleeping on the side throughout the night. A hard pillow at the back will aid in maintaining this position. In the author's experience an excellent way to fix the habit of sleeping on the side is to sleep on a very narrow bed, such as half of a boudoir couch, so that any attempt to turn on the back without being fully awake is likely to result in falling out of bed. Even in sleep the instinct of self-preservation seems to be quite strong, so that the unconscious back turn is soon discarded.

Surgical treatment to harden the soft palate by means of injection has given relief from snoring in some cases, though the treatment is not regarded as entirely satisfactory, and in any case it is not striking at the real cause.

Control of the Throat

The best discussion of snoring that the author has been able to find is in a little book, *How to Stop Snoring,* by David Harwich. His basic proposition is that the soft palate, while it actually produces the noise in snoring, is not alone responsible, but must have the active cooperation of neighboring parts of the throat. It is for this reason he says that surgery or other treatments directed at the soft palate alone have had so little success in controlling snoring. He suggests that the snorer watch in a mirror the parts of the throat in what he calls the snore chamber back of the soft palate, including the base of the tongue, and see them taking position for a voluntary snore produced while the snorer is awake. These parts in the snore chamber he contends are the ones that must be controlled if snoring is to be stopped.

Since all these parts are of course moved by muscles and can change position only by contraction of these muscles, Mr. Harwich emphasizes the importance of learning to relax the muscles of the throat and neighboring parts and keep them in this condition during sleep. He gives detailed instructions for accomplishing this purpose, leaning heavily on autosuggestion.

Mr. Harwich is unquestionably on solid ground when he further contends that snoring is the result simply of a bad habit which has by some chance become fixed in these throat muscles, and that its cure, in the absence of pathological conditions, depends on breaking this habit. Recognizing that for the snorer to oppose and overcome a habit by his own will power while he is unconscious in sleep is a pretty large order, Mr. Harwich advises that in addition to carrying out other instructions the snorer arrange to have another person wake him when he begins to snore. When wide awake he must repeat the procedures for throat control before he goes to sleep again. By persistence in this program the snoring habit is eventually broken.

Soldiers on the battle line, when they have a chance to sleep, usually sleep too soundly to be disturbed by a comrade's snoring. But in a training barracks one loud snorer can seriously disturb the sleep of a whole group. During the war the disturbance became so serious in one group that something had to be done about it. The snorer was well liked and always disposed to be cooperative. So his barracks mates told him the situation and secured his approval of their plan to cure him. They were to take turns in waiting by his bunk throughout the night until he was cured. Each watcher kept in hand a heavy roll of old newspapers, and when a snore started he gave the snorer a sharp whack across the hips. This produced a loud report and a rude shock to the snorer, but caused no pain or injury. Only a few nights of this treatment were needed for a complete and permanent cure.

If one is to make a broadly intelligent approach to the question of a cure for snoring, there are a few fundamental facts which must be considered. First, no one snores when he is awake, no matter how he breathes, through mouth or nose or both, vigorously or quietly, and no matter what condition may prevail in his air passages. Yet anyone can, by deliberate purpose, produce a snore when he is awake, equally independent of manner of breathing or condition of air passages. This indicates that the immediate cause of snoring is some change in the air passages brought about by muscles which can be activated by voluntary conscious control. This being true, what we have to do in order to cure snoring is to find a way of controlling the unconscious activation of these snoring muscles.

You Can Control Yourself When You Sleep. Can a person learn to control his activities while he is unconscious in sleep? *Fortunately* *for the snorer and his friends, the answer is an unequivocal yes.* One of the mysteries of sleep is that while unconscious and apparently entirely unaware of our surroundings, we are nevertheless ready to respond to certain occurrences or conditions, by waking if this is necessary, but in some cases while remaining soundly asleep. Perhaps the most familiar and universal example of a response while asleep is in the changing of position in bed. When discomfort arises from lying in one position the sleeper turns to another without waking. Students of sleep have found that this occurs many times during a night of normal sleep. And not only are these changes of position made without waking, but the sleeper goes further and takes good care that he does not roll himself out of bed when he changes position. Successful training of a sleeper to awake in response to a special signal is seen in the telegrapher who sleeps through the clicking of all the keys until his own signal comes and then is instantly wide awake, also in the mother who sleeps through all kinds of noise until she hears her baby's cry.

Probably the closest parallel to our snoring problem is in the toilet training of young children. Babies habitually empty bowels or bladder on impulse, whether awake or asleep, without any restraint whatever. They must be taught to control these impulses, not only when awake, but equally well when asleep. The older child's unconscious awareness results from his having learned to inhibit the natural spontaneous action, and to awake, so that he can go to the toilet. With persistent training this ability is acquired by all normal children.

A further fact to be recognized is that the activity of these snoring muscles is only a useless habit, formed in most cases by some unrecognized chance influence which led to breathing with various parts of the air passages held by their muscles in the snoring position. So the snoring problem narrows down to the problem of finding a sound psychological procedure for training the mind to oppose and suppress this undesirable habit.

The first essential in breaking any habit is to prevent the exercise of the objectionable activity. In waking habits this can be done by will power, though various aids to will power can make the task much easier. But, in snoring, will power cannot be used, because while we are unconscious in sleep will power is not in action.

So we have to fall back on reflex action, which does not depend on consciousness. The greater part of the body's activities are in fact controlled by reflexes even when we are fully conscious, and when we are asleep all activities of the body are reflex, such as breathing, heart beats, movements of the digestive organs, even the change of position in bed. A reflex may be defined as an order for activity sent to a muscle or gland from a nerve center in response to some impression received through the senses, this order being sent without the intervention of the conscious mind. True reflexes are not learned, being inborn. But psychologists now speak of conditioned reflexes, meaning learned reflexes. They are in reality habits which have become so fixed that they act like the inborn reflexes. This means that it is possible for us to form a habit while we are conscious which will exert its control over our actions even while we are asleep.

So in order to stop snoring, which is a habit, we must form an opposing habit which will be strong enough to assert itself as a conditioned reflex, in this way becoming effective even during sleep. Habits are formed by repetition of the activity, just as they are broken by preventing the activity. This means that in forming the stopping habit which is to cure snoring we will also be preventing the snoring and thus weakening the snoring habit. This double effect will greatly shorten the task of making the new habit stronger than the old one.

Habit forming is a type of training, and in all training there are two stimulants that can be used to increase the effects of repetition. These are rewards and punishments. Both are very commonly used in the training of children, and they are the main dependence in the training of animals. Training the subconscious mind would seem to be closely akin to the training of animals. Can we then use rewards or punishments to aid in establishing the anti-snoring habit?

Mr. Harwich in his book emphasizes the fact that the repetition of a required ritual by the awakened snorer before he is free to return to sleep serves to attach a sort of penalty to the snoring. Recalling the incident related above of the snoring soldier, it is clear that not only the repeated awakenings to stop the snoring, but also the unpleasant method of the waking were both effective factors in the cure. Reward in these cases is not so apparent, but the snorer's desire to be rid of the habit can offer him a very effective final reward.

Summary: Aid for the Victims

While we have now the essential principles on which a cure for snoring can be based, a cure may take a little time. Fortunately there are some means of self-defense meantime which are available to the snorer's victims. Perhaps the best is a pair of tight-fitting ear plugs. The homemade plugs described in Chapter Seven of this book will be found effective.

Some persons find it possible to become inured to snoring just as they do to other noises, though it is to be hoped that few will reach the stage of the legendary old lady who when her husband was away found it impossible to sleep except by having her daughters take turns throughout the night in grinding the family's old-fashioned coffee mill.

The author has for some years taken his afternoon nap to the accompaniment of a noise machine devised from an old electric fan placed in contact with his bedstead. The effect on his ears is about the equivalent of a passing freight train and fully submerges any ordinary noises that occur about the house. So far as he can judge the noise of this machine softened by ear plugs does not delay the coming of sleep or reduce its restfulness. Perhaps a similar device to be turned on when snoring starts would serve the double purpose of eventually breaking the snorer's habit while in the meantime serving to submerge the intermittent noise of the snores for the benefit of the snorer's bed mate.

16. How your breath can regulate your brain

CO_2 Used as Anesthetic

For more than a hundred years it has been known that carbon dioxide will produce the deep sleep called anesthesia. It was in fact the first substance used in modern surgery to produce the kind of sleep needed for surgical operations. When the English doctor, Henry Hickman, in the early part of the last century, made his revolutionary experiments in surgical anesthesia, the animals on which he operated were put to sleep by causing them to breathe the carbon dioxide from their own breaths. His experiments were highly successful. His incisions caused little bleeding and the wounds healed rapidly. In America, many years later, drugs were introduced that were more suitable for surgery than carbon dioxide, principally because of their longer-lasting effects. In recent years, however, carbon dioxide has been extensively used to produce a brief therapeutic sleep used in the treatment of mental patients.

As Dr. Hickman used it, and as it is now used in treating mental patients, where the carbon dioxide is drawn from a tank and breathed in high concentrations, its effect is very similar to that of the commonly used sleep-producing drugs, except that its action is very brief and entirely harmless. All the common sleep-producing drugs produce their effects by what may be truthfully called a poisoning of the nervous system, especially the brain. Many of these drugs produce a cumulative effect, so that their continued use may cause permanent damage to the nerves or the brain. All of these drugs are chemicals which are not naturally found in the body, and they produce effects which do not occur in the body's natural processes.

By contrast, the effects of carbon dioxide are natural effects, and they are produced by only slight increases of carbon dioxide. They occur in the bodies of all of us every day, usually without our being aware of them, certainly without our being aware of the connection between the effects and the carbon dioxide content of our bodies. For want of a better name we may call these the hormone effects of carbon dioxide.

CO_2 As a Regulatory Hormone

It will, no doubt, come as a surprise to most of us to have carbon dioxide referred to as a hormone. But physiologists are now giving authoritative recognition to many such effects of carbon dioxide in our bodies. Best and Taylor in their textbook of human physiology, *The Living Body* (fourth edition, page 403), state the matter plainly: "The term hormone is not, however, restricted to the secretions of the ductless glands. Any substance formed by a tissue of the body and carried in the blood stream to act as an excitant to some other tissue or organ may be called a hormone. Thus, . . . even carbon dioxide, since it is carried by the blood and acts upon the respiratory and vasomotor centers, comes into this category." As a group, the hormones are the principal regulators of the body's life processes. And carbon dioxide is one of the most important and most continuously active of the entire group.

As is the case with other hormones, an increase in the amount of carbon dioxide above that naturally contained in the fluids and tissues of the body can be used to bring about very noticeable and often surprising results. When very slightly increased, carbon dioxide acts as a sedative, quieting activity or excitement in the nervous system, including the brain as well as what are commonly called the nerves. This quieting or relaxing effect extends to the muscles as well as to the nerves, because muscles act only as they are stimulated by impulses brought to them by the nerves. A striking example of this sedative effect is seen when breathing carbon dioxide stops the spasmodic contractions of the diaphragm which we call hiccups.

A moderate increase of the carbon dioxide in the body tends to bring on drowsiness, which under favorable conditions may lead to sleep. This sleep-producing effect is of special interest because it can be so easily brought about by merely reducing the volume of breathing. Breathing, when we give it no attention, is unconsciously regulated to retain only a limited amount of carbon dioxide in the blood, but when we wish, a change can be made in the breathing which will bring the carbon dioxide up to the drowsiness level. The special advantages of using self-produced carbon dioxide as an aid to sleep will be pointed out in the following paragraphs.

Always Available, Always Safe

It is important to note that the anesthetic effect of carbon dioxide cannot be produced by controlled breathing, because when consciousness is lost, control is also lost, and breathing automatically goes back to normal. Consequently the use of carbon dioxide from controlled breathing as a means of inducing sleep has a 100 per cent safety factor not possessed by any hypnotic drug.

The use of carbon dioxide as a sleep aid instead of hypnotic drugs has a distinct advantage in the way of convenience because it does not have to be taken in advance of the time when its sleep-producing effect is desired. When retained in the lungs it is carried almost instantly through the blood stream to all parts of the body, so that it begins its relaxing and quieting effects on the nerves and muscles immediately. Drugs taken by mouth are absorbed more slowly and cannot take effect so promptly. The effects of many hypnotic drugs taken by mouth are not felt until after an hour or more

A further advantage of carbon dioxide as a sleep aid is that it is always immediately available without previous planning or preparation. Since a large excess of it is being constantly produced by the body, no trip is required to a doctor for a prescription or to the drug store for its purchase. This means, too, that there is no expense. It is, literally, "as free as the air we breathe." In fact, it is even freer. We do have to breathe the air. Carbon dioxide we have already within us, and we only need to keep it in by not breathing it out.

As perhaps the greatest of all its advantages over hypnotic drugs, carbon dioxide can be trusted as perfectly safe because of the special nature of its action on the nerve cells of the body. The best consensus of opinion among physiologists is that it has no poisoning or paralyzing effect on the cells of the brain or nerves, but only has a blanketing effect, so that the natural action of the cells is merely impeded or held back temporarily. The difference between carbon dioxide and the usual hypnotic drugs is something like the difference in a city between a snow storm and a period of smog. The snow hinders operations, but it soon melts and activities go on unhindered. The after-effects of smog may be felt over a long period.

An extremely important advantage is that the dose of carbon dioxide when it is taken by the method of controlled breathing is self-regulating. No over-dosage is possible, either by accident or by deliberate intention. As soon as a sufficient amount has been accumulated in the body to produce sleep, the voluntary effect by which breathing had been reduced necessarily ceases. Automatic, unconscious control of breathing then takes over and eliminates within a few minutes all the excess of carbon dioxide except the small increase which is natural to sleep.

Controlled Breathing Sleep Is Natural Sleep

Sleep induced by controlled breathing is natural sleep. The increase of carbon dioxide merely serves to overcome the obstacles which have prevented the onset of sleep, and when this has been accomplished, the increase is at once reduced to normal levels by automatic breathing. The blanketing effect which was needed to quiet the nerve cells then ceases, and sleep goes on under perfectly natural conditions. The commonly-used, long-acting hypnotic drugs, such as the barbiturates, may produce extended poisoning effects, some through many hours, so that the sleep which they produce is really a doped sleep, a sort of unnatural stupor, and not really restful, restorative sleep. In marked contrast to this prolonged stupor, the action of carbon dioxide is merely to initiate sleep. Then it is quickly and automatically removed, while sleep continues with its natural restorative action unhampered even by the mild effect of carbon dioxide which induced it.

Compared with most of the hypnotics in common use carbon dioxide may seem too mild in its effect. But this, too, is a decided advantage. Because of this mildness it cannot be used as a pain reliever to cover up the symptoms of what may be a serious illness, thus delaying proper treatment. The dosage of carbon dioxide which it is possible to accumulate in the body by controlled breathing will not produce sleep when pain is present or when there is any serious bodily or mental disturbance. And this constitutes a still further advantage, for it requires that noise and various bodily discomforts must be controlled, and that the mind must be calmed and freed of disturbing thoughts, thus paving the way for the continuance of sleep under conditions which will make it really restful.

Repeated use of carbon dioxide from controlled breathing is both practical and safe. It can be used several times in the same night if needed, or even for the purpose of securing a short daytime nap. This feature is especially important for persons who are inclined to wake too early in the morning. Carbon dioxide will give them the hour or two of extra sleep they need to put an edge on their energy as they face the day's duties. And even when used late in the night carbon dioxide leaves no hangover of dullness to destroy the value of the extra sleep.

Because carbon dioxide is one of the body's own natural regulators, because an over-dosage cannot be produced by controlled breathing, and because it is so quickly eliminated from the body through the lungs, making its time of action very short, there is no tendency to develop a tolerance for it as there is with hypnotic drugs. The need for constantly increasing the dose, which is a marked characteristic of the hypnotic drugs commonly used, is completely absent. In fact, the tendency is rather toward smaller dosages. This is partly due to the fact that as confidence is developed in the effectiveness of carbon dioxide, the fear of wakefulness, which is one of the greatest hindrances to sleep, is lost and no longer needs to be overcome. Also a habit of going to sleep under the influence of the breathing procedures is gradually developed—a conditioned reflex—and this still further reduces the need for the sleep-inducing effect of carbon dioxide. The need for the extra push into sleep which carbon dioxide can give will, of course, vary with bodily and mental conditions, but the dosage is always automatically limited to the actual need, and this on the average will almost invariably be found to decrease over an extended period of use.

Seventeen Years of Successful Use

For the past seventeen years I have been using controlled breathing as a sleep-inducer whenever sleep did not come promptly, securing by this means the aid of increased carbon dioxide. Probably I have used this controlled breathing procedure a total number of times equal to an average of once a day for the entire period and I have never been able to detect even the slightest undesirable or unpleasant effect. Now at the age of eighty-six, I am in good health, with near-perfect digestion and few aches or pains, with no slowing of my typing, and my mental alertness seemingly unimpaired. This prolonged vigor I attribute largely to the adequate sleep which I have always managed to get, and which I am now continuing to ensure by the use of controlled breathing.

Sleep is not, of course, a cure for all of our bodily ills. It cannot set a broken bone, but it can materially hasten its healing. It cannot remove a diseased appendix, but it can at least hasten recovery from the operation. Sleep is our best means of strengthening nature's own powers of recuperation, and for these there is no substitute, either in surgery or in medicine.

The recuperative power of sleep is by no means limited to the body. Many tests have shown that the body can continue to function reasonably well without sleep for a much longer time than the mind can. It may even be that the main reason why sleep is necessary is to give the brain an opportunity to rest. Our heart muscles rest between beats. Our breathing muscles rest between breaths. Even our voluntary muscles, if not allowed to rest between exertions, will go only so far until they call a halt and demand rest. But our consciousness, which is maintained by the activities of the brain, can take no interim rests. As long as we are awake our minds must remain continuously on the alert. Many years ago Dr. George Crile, the surgeon who founded the Cleveland Clinic, put the brain's special need for sleep bluntly by saying, "The brain cannot work continuously, but a reversible process is necessary at regular intervals to restore it. This process in the higher centers is called sleep. The more intense the activation, the more needed is sleep. The brain is the only organ that sleeps conspicuously. Of great significance is the fact that the entire man spends one-third of his time waiting for the brain to restore itself."

Recharging the Brain

Doctor Crile likened the brain to the electric battery of a car, its effective action being maintained only by recharging. Fortunately a car's battery can be recharged while the car is running, without being disconnected. But our brains must be disconnected for recharge, and this disconnection can be accomplished only in sleep. Dr. Nathaniel Kleitman describes this disconnection as a "functional deafferentiation of the cerebral cortex," and he considers it to be the immediate cause of sleep, the deafferentiation itself being brought about by reduction of the nervous impulses which stimulate the wakefulness center of the brain. Controlled

breathing is successful in bringing sleep because directly or indirectly it reduces this nervous stimulation of the wakefulness
center.

Men who service car batteries will tell you that if a battery is
to give long and satisfactory service it should be maintained as
nearly as possible in a fully charged condition. A battery continuously or frequently used to a state of exhaustion can be expected to give poor service and have a shortened life. Our mental
activities are just as certainly dependent on an alert condition in
our brains as the electrical equipment of a car is dependent on
a full charge in the battery, and we can expect to pay an un-
welcome price if in either case we fail to assure prompt and proper
recharging.

For those who are interested in the physiological processes by
which carbon dioxide induces sleep, two outstanding features may
be mentioned as being clearly in evidence. Too little is known at
present about the nature of sleep itself and about the various
phenomena which surround its approach to permit any complete
enumeration of all the ways in which it may be influenced by an
increase of carbon dioxide in the blood and tissues. But two basic
factors in the approach of sleep are definitely known to be strongly
promoted by carbon dioxide. These are a reduction in the body's
internal temperature and a quieting of the activities of the entire
nervous system.

Dr. Gudmund Magnusson, prominent Danish psychiatrist, in a
lecture on sleep at the Fourth International Congress on Mental
Health, strongly emphasized what he called "vegetative sleep pre-
paredness," consisting of certain changes which take place unconsciously in the body to prepare the way for sleep. One of the
most important of these he said is a change in body temperature,
the skin becoming warmer while at the same time a fall in the
internal temperature of the body occurs. This dual and opposite
effect is caused by a dilation of the small blood vessels of the skin
and especially of the fingers and toes. This brings an increased
flow of blood to the surface of the body where its heat is rapidly

lost to the air thus warming the surface but rapidly lowering the internal temperature. Laboratory studies showed, Dr. Magnusson said, that this rise in skin temperature occurs before a person actually falls asleep, indicating he said that it is a "necessary precursor or foundation for sleep."

Until quite recently it was believed that an increase of carbon dioxide in the blood would cause contraction of the peripheral blood vessels, such as those of the skin and fingers, and it is true that when a mixture of carbon dioxide in air is breathed such contraction does occur. But Altschule and Sulzbach, working in the medical laboratory at Harvard, showed that the contraction of the peripheral blood vessels is not caused by the carbon dioxide but that it is a nervous reflex effect arising from the increased activity of the breathing muscles in their effort to throw off the increased carbon dioxide. When artificial respiration was used, with the breathing muscles inactive, and air containing carbon dioxide was breathed, it produced instead a dilation of the blood vessels of the skin and limbs. These investigators reported that they found it possible, when administering carbon dioxide under these conditions, to increase the blood flow through the fingers as much as 500 per cent.

The point to be noted here is that when the body's own production of carbon dioxide is accumulated in the body by means of controlled breathing the activity of the breathing muscles is not increased but substantially decreased, thus leaving the blood vessels of the skin and extremities free from reflex nervous control. When thus freed they show a very marked dilation in response to the effect of carbon dioxide, with a corresponding increase in the blood flow to the body surfaces. In this way heat is rapidly lost and the internal temperature of the body reduced. This furnishes what Dr. Magnusson called a "foundation for sleep."

The effect of carbon dioxide in dilating the blood vessels of the skin is strikingly illustrated by the late Dr. W. B. Cannon in his famous book, *The Wisdom of the Body*. He points out that if a person takes a bath in water at 84 degrees Fahrenheit he feels cold and shivers, but if he takes a bath at the same temperature in carbonated water (water in which carbon dioxide has been dissolved) he does not shiver nor feel cold. This is because his skin is kept warm by the greatly increased flow of blood which results from dilation of the blood vessels by the carbon dioxide absorbed from the water.

Your Drowsiness Temperature Level

As pointed out by Dr. Magnusson, dilation of the blood vessels of the skin causes a loss of heat and a lowering of the body's internal temperature. Dr. Nathaniel Kleitman in his book *Sleep and Wakefulness,* goes very thoroughly into the relation of the body temperature to sleep, and his conclusion is that each person probably has a "drowsiness temperature level," above which it is easy for him to remain awake and below which he has an increasing inclination to fall asleep, this referring of course to internal body temperature, not to skin temperature.

Beginning in early childhood, Dr. Kleitman found, the body tends to develop a daily cycle of temperature change, the highest point coming during the customary hours of wakefulness and the lowest during the usual hours of sleep. This cycle persists over a considerable period when an effort is made to change the hours of sleep from night to day, and it accounts for much of the difficulty that night workers have in sleeping during the daytime. Their higher internal temperature resists their best efforts to obtain sleep. When a person sleeps at his accustomed time, this habitual low point of his internal temperature becomes a highly effective aid to him in going to sleep. When this habitual cycle of internal temperature hinders the coming of sleep, controlled breathing affords an ideal means of overcoming it, because the increased carbon dioxide dilates the blood vessels of the skin and causes a loss of the body's heat.

While a popular idea prevails that when we are warm we get sleepy, when we are cold we wake up, this is true only for external body temperature, the temperature of the skin. There are nerves which tell us of the skin temperature, but none to tell us when the internal temperature of the body falls or rises, so that we are not directly conscious of these internal changes. Under ordinary conditions, of course, there are only slight changes in the internal temperature, though the skin temperature may vary many degrees, making us acutely aware of the change. The internal temperatures produce their effect, however, whether we are aware of them or not. It is significant in this connection that when a person is freezing to death, with internal temperatures extremely reduced, the urge to sleep becomes irresistible. In modern surgery it has been found that the lowering of body temperature will greatly reduce the amount of anesthetic required.

CO_2 as Nerve-quieter. It is now fully recognized by the medical profession that carbon dioxide is a safe and effective "depressant" of the nervous system. These terms mean that it can be depended upon to slow the activities and decrease the excitability of the brain and the nerves without producing undesirable "side effects." While carbon dioxide has a quieting effect on other parts of the nervous system, it produces an exactly opposite effect on the respiratory center of the brain, so that it is now accepted in medical practice as one of the most effective respiratory stimulants.

Because of the recognition of its usefulness both for quieting the nervous system and for stimulating breathing, tanks of carbon dioxide, often in combination with oxygen, have become a standard gas available from all medical gas suppliers. It would be possible to use carbon dioxide from the patient's body in many cases just as effectively as from the tank, except that it is easier to measure the dosage by turning a valve than by regulating the patient's breathing. In an increasing number of cases, however, where only moderate dosage is required and where exact control is not needed, the carbon dioxide in the patient's breath is being utilized by having him breathe into a paper bag and then rebreathe the expired air, which of course contains a considerable percentage of carbon dioxide. A rubber tube of proper length may be substituted for the paper bag, and will give better control for the dosage of carbon dioxide. This procedure has proved very useful in treating the nervous spasms of the diaphragm which we call hiccups.

As an aid in diagnosis it is sometimes desirable to decrease the amount of carbon dioxide in the patient's blood, because the resulting increase in alkalinity of the blood heightens the activity of the nervous system. In this way the brain can be stimulated by over-breathing, enabling the physician to diagnose abnormalities in brain function.

In recording the electrical activity of the brain by the electroencephalograph it has become standard practice to require the patient to over-breathe. This heightens the activity of the brain, making the abnormal activity evident in the electroencephalograph. When this stimulating effect on the nervous system is desired, it is always secured by having the patient increase his breathing, because the voluntary increase of breathing is much simpler and easier than any artificial substitute could be, although the same effect can be produced in an iron lung when it is operated too rapidly.

In recent years a great deal of time has been devoted by various scientists to the study of the effects of carbon dioxide on nerve action. One of the most thorough and exhaustive experimental studies was that of Lorente de Nó, working at the Rockefeller Institute in New York. He found that in order to maintain excised nerve in normal condition for any considerable length of time it must be surrounded by an atmosphere containing five per cent of carbon dioxide, and that the percentage of carbon dioxide in the atmosphere surrounding the nerve could be increased up to a full one hundred per cent without any appreciable damage to the nerve. In an atmosphere of five per cent carbon dioxide he found that the ability of the nerve to perform work was increased, but that its resistance to excitement or stimulation was much greater than when the nerve was in ordinary air, which contains only a small fraction of one per cent of carbon dioxide. It was also shown by these researches of de Nó that carbon dioxide exerts an effective control over the spontaneous or spasmodic activity of the nerve, and that it has a quieting effect which is independent of and in addition to the quieting which could be expected to result from the lowering of the nerve's alkalinity.

The quieting effect of carbon dioxide upon the nerves is supported by the results of many other investigators. Among these is Dr. L. J. Meduna's recent discovery that carbon dioxide reduces the secretion of the thyroid hormone, thus quieting the nerves indirectly. This hormone, it seems, largely controls the speed with which all the processes of living take place. So when carbon dioxide reduces thyroid secretion the effect is to slow all bodily activities and processes.

Dr. Hornell Hart in his book, *Autoconditioning,* describes a method of bringing sleep by means of autosuggestion given during self-induced hypnosis. Since the procedure proposed for self-hypnosis places great emphasis on extreme relaxation of the muscles, a person following this procedure can hardly fail to slow up the action of the breathing muscles, thus producing the respiratory acidosis which Dr. Kety's experiments in Philadelphia (see Chapter One) indicate is probably a necessary condition of sleep. Dr. Hart adds that in his own experience, after relaxing on his back, he goes to sleep best by turning over and lying face down. He does not explain how this change of the body position helps, but in all probability it is by placing the weight of the body on the chest and abdomen and thus reducing the movements of breathing. When added to the effect of relaxation this face-down position easily increases the carbon dioxide in the blood enough to significantly aid the coming of sleep. So it would seem that an increase of carbon dioxide in the blood plays an important if unconscious part, even in Dr. Hart's method of inducing sleep.

Under normal waking conditions when the carbon dioxide of the blood is increased the respiratory center of the brain responds quickly with an increase of breathing. Just why a similar response does not occur during sleep or with the approach of sleep is not definitely known. Apparently the respiratory center develops a tolerance for carbon dioxide, probably as part of the vegetative (unconscious) preparation for sleep referred to by Dr. Magnusson, so that the carbon dioxide of the blood can be increased moderately without the usual increase of breathing. Experiments by Dr. Robin and his associates at Harvard Medical School led to the conclusion that this change of response from the respiratory center is not due to a change in the constituents of the blood, but that it is brought about through the agency of the nervous system.

Summary: Sleep's Enemy—Nerve Activity

Experience has taught physicians that if the coming of sleep is to be made certain and prompt, it is not enough merely to provide conditions favorable to sleep. In all cases where the lack of sleep is serious enough to be harmful, physicians most likely will prescribe a hypnotic drug, or at least a sedative, in order to secure its direct action in controlling the brain and nerves, because they recognize that nervous activity is the outstanding enemy of sleep, whether this activity has its source in the body, in the brain, or in outside conditions.

Since carbon dioxide accumulated in the body through reduced breathing has all the advantages described in the first part of this chapter, it is on every count much to be preferred to the barbiturates and other sleep-producing drugs, either those advertised for self-treatment or those obtainable on prescription.

17. How safe are sedatives, sleeping pills and tranquilizers?

Danger of Barbiturate Addiction

The curative and restorative effects of sleep are so great that doctors have always felt justified in using drugs when necessary to secure its benefits to their patients. Until the beginning of this century their main dependence was on opiates, principally morphine, codeine, and heroin. But the danger of addiction to these drugs was so great, the effects of addiction were so terrible, and to cure it was so difficult, that the doctors were only too glad to welcome the barbiturates when they were discovered in 1903. The use of opiates was dropped except for the control of intense pain, and the new compounds of barbituric acid came into general use for the production of sleep.

At first it was believed that there was little if any danger of addiction in the use of the barbiturate drugs, and as long as they were used only on a physician's prescription in small doses and for short periods the danger of addiction was slight. But when barbiturates are used continuously for any length of time the patient develops a tolerance for the drug, so that the dose has to be continually increased to produce the original effect, and this continued increase will at last bring on addiction. This term addiction means that changes have been produced in the patient's body which make the presence of the drug necessary to maintain the ordinary processes of living, and failure to get the drug causes serious disturbances. It is a fact that in confirmed cases of barbiturate addiction failure to get the drugs may cause convulsions and even death.

It was only after barbiturates had been in use twenty or thirty years that physicians began to realize the serious danger of addiction. In this time a considerable number of their patients had reached the stage where they could not do without the drug. This was especially likely to happen where unlimited refilling of a prescription was permitted. With increasing numbers of addicts a large and profitable bootleg market also developed. The drugs can be produced cheaply, and a few states still permit their sale without a prescription. With a ready source of supply, and in the absence of federal regulation, the drugs can be bootlegged in comparative safety. Mail-order houses and unscrupulous druggists have entered this market. The figures for total barbiturate sales are almost too large to be comprehended. Allowing one-tenth of a gram, the usual dose to produce sleep, one pound of the drugs will make more than four thousand doses, and nearly a million pounds are made and sold each year in the United States.

The clandestine sale of barbiturate drugs was greatly increased when users discovered that in combination with benzedrine they act, not as sedatives or hypnotics, but as exciting stimulants, producing a real intoxication. Their effects on the brain are variable, making behavior unpredictable. The addict may pick a fight with a friend or break up the furniture, yet remember nothing of the occurrence. A morphine addict often keeps his job and lives almost normally. But the barbiturate addict neglects his appearance and his duties, creates needless disturbances, and soon loses his job and his friends. Barbiturate addiction is more difficult to cure and more dangerous to life than addiction to opiates or any other drug. Doctors of the U. S. drug addiction hospital at Lexington, Kentucky, say that an opiate addict can safely be taken off his drug within a week, but a barbiturate addict requires two or three weeks or even longer. To effect an apparent cure of the addiction is also more difficult, requiring months. And cases of return to the drug after cure are frequent.

The barbiturate addict's memory is hazy, so that he is apt to forget how much of the drug he has taken and to repeat the dose, or even to take a handful of the pills, causing a sleep that ends in death. Barbiturates greatly increase the user's liability to accidents, including automobile accidents. Airplane pilots are grounded for a month after using the drugs even temporarily. Barbiturates and alcohol are what doctors call synergistic drugs. Each increases the effect of the other. Like alcohol and opium, barbiturates are deceptive. The user does not suspect that he is approaching addiction until it is too late to escape. The only safe plan is to leave them strictly alone except under the close and continuous supervision of an experienced and careful physician.

In very small doses the barbiturates act merely as sedatives, and being inexpensive, they are still widely used for this purpose. In larger doses the barbiturates are very effective in bringing sleep, though for many people this sleep is far from refreshing. They awake feeling drowsy, often with dizziness and headache. Even when such symptoms are absent mental and memory tests usually show that the patient is below par in his mental processes. Basically, all the barbiturates are brain depressants. The different types vary only in the speed and duration of their effects, which are produced by inhibiting the oxidation of glucose. Patients vary so much in their response that exact dosage is difficult to determine. The doctor must of course make the dose large enough to guarantee sleep. For a patient with defective kidneys or a damaged liver this may easily be a serious overdosage.

Now, something more than fifty years after the doctors gave such a ready welcome to the barbiturates, they have given an equal welcome to a class of drugs commonly called tranquilizers. While these drugs are not classed as hypnotics, or even sedatives, many doctors prescribe them for the purpose of affording sleep, and the claim is made that they afford sleep only because they reduce anxiety, and that consequently the sleep they produce is natural sleep. But the effect of these drugs on the brain lasts for several hours, often outlasting the sleep. Consequently the patient sleeps in a doped condition, and sleeps because he is doped.

Tranquilizers

The truth is that the tranquilizer drugs are so new that no one yet knows what their effects are or how the drugs should be classed. As Dr. Felix of the National Institutes of Health puts it, they do something to the brain, and we don't know all that they do, or even where they do it. The first of these drugs to be introduced in the U. S. came from India, the root of a shrub with the botanical name *Rauwolfia serpentina,* and it was at first prescribed, not as a tranquilizer, but to reduce blood pressure. Dr. R. W. Wilkins, of Boston, noticed that Rauwolfia quieted some excitable patients to whom he was giving it for reduction of blood pressure. His report of this effect started its use as a tranquilizer. This drug is used in two forms, a whole root preparation sold as Raudixin, and a refinement of the active principle, reserpine, sold largely under the trade name Serpasil. A synthetic drug, chlorpromazine, produced in France and sold as Thorazine was introduced in the United States about the same time as Rauwolfia. It was found to produce very similar effects on the brain. Soon afterward American chemists synthesized a third drug, meprobamate, which while chemically different produced similar effects. It has been sold as Miltown and Equanil.

The drugs of these three classes vary somewhat in their tranquilizing effects, and even more in their so-called "side effects," effects which are usually undesirable, and may even be dangerous to susceptible patients. Sometimes there is a complete reversal of the expected quieting effect, the patient becoming instead violently excited. Unfortunately there is so far no means of determining beforehand what the effect will be. Consequently the taking of tranquilizers must be classed as at best a "calculated risk" on the part of the patient. Authorities are now warning users of tranquilizers not to take alcoholic drinks if they are planning to drive a car or to operate machinery. The two drugs are synergistic in their effects on the brain. After taking a tranquilizer, even a small amount of whiskey can make a man so drunk that he does not know what he is doing.

In experiments on mice, and in some human patients, the tranquilizers have shown characteristics of tolerance and addiction very similar to those of alcohol and barbiturates. All are drugs which change the natural activities of the brain. These activities are so delicately balanced, and the brain is so delicately organized, that all drugs which affect its activities must be used with great caution and their use closely supervised by a physician with special knowledge and adequate experience. Any other use, especially if continued over a considerable period of time, may cause possibly irreparable damage.

Loss of "Aliveness"

The enormous sale of tranquilizing drugs has caused a large number of pharmaceutical firms to enter the market with similar drugs under their own trade names, so that now there are more than forty of these trade names in use. Practically all of the drugs sold under these various names are derivatives or relatives of the original three classes, and their effects do not vary greatly. They may dull the ability of the mind to imagine, to foresee, to think ahead. Under their influence a business executive may lose the ability to discern in advance the conditions which his business will have to meet. Persons engaged in routine or mechanical tasks lose the urge to accuracy and efficiency, since they no longer realize the effects that must come from carelessness and delay. Recent animal experiments seem to indicate that tranquilizing drugs interfere with learning ability, and also erase knowledge gained by previous experience, including highly important conditioned reflexes. The total of these effects is to take the edge off a person's aliveness.

The drug houses, realizing the possibilities of the market, have lost no opportunity to stimulate the sale of the tranquilizers, bringing advertising pressure to bear not only on physicians, who must prescribe the drugs, but also on the lay public, so that now a high percentage of the doctor's patients come to him demanding that he prescribe these drugs. The doctor's natural caution has been largely overcome by the claims of the manufacturers that these drugs are perfectly safe and entirely harmless. The result is that a large proportion of all prescriptions now being written call for or contain tranquilizers, with sale of the tablets now being counted in billions.

The tranquilizing drugs undoubtedly have a great field of useful service in the treatment of the violently insane, and even in the arrest of incipient insanity, fields which have been so dramatically set forth by Paul de Kruif's book *Man Against Insanity*. But there is a vast difference between the intelligent and careful prescribing of drugs for the treatment of insanity and the casual issuance of "peace of mind pills" in response to the desire, which is natural to every person, to have life made easy, to have the rough places smoothed over. To be able to substitute drugs for electro-shock and lobotomy in the treatment of insane patients is no doubt a great gain. But to prescribe brain-depressant drugs for the everyday problems of people with normal minds, instead of seeking rational solutions, is certainly a great mistake.

Primitive man, living in caves and threatened principally by prowling animals, could shut out his fears and worries at night by means of fires and barricades. Modern man's fears and worries are largely intangible and internal. No material means can afford freedom and security from them. Consequently men are continually searching for internal, subjective, mental barriers against their fears and worries. But to deaden the brain so that it loses its awareness of the besetting worries is exactly equivalent to the act of the traditional ostrich which was said to stick its head in the sand, in this way putting its pursuers out of sight. Primitive man was at least wise enough not to block the entrance of his cave to the point where he suffocated in the smoke of his fire. It remains to

Summary: Escape, Yes—By Dope, No.

Today many of us are obliged to live under high tension. Intervals of escape from this tension are necessary to health of both mind and body. Various avenues of escape have been recommended, such as hobbies, sports, travel, and religion. No doubt each of these has its place. But sleep remains the most perfect escape. The man who can be sure of going to sleep when he needs sleep has the perfect antidote to tensions and worries. But if in his efforts to get sleep he resorts to drugs which undermine the foundations of both physical and mental health he will eventually find that he has paid too high a price for his surcease from worry.

The many advantages of using carbon dioxide accumulated in the body by means of reduced breathing, in place of the commonly used drugs for producing sleep, were described in detail in chapter 16. For those who have not yet begun the use of sleeping pills or tranquilizers these outstanding advantages should bring a firm resolve to pass up the drugs in favor of this better and safer method. For those who have already begun the use of drugs, and have not yet carried it too far, the procedures outlined in this book offer a simple and practical means of escape.

In most cases it is better not to break off the use of drugs abruptly, but instead to reduce the dosage gradually. At first a slight reduction should be made, with the breathing procedures used as a supplement. After a short time, when sleep begins to come easily, a further reduction of the drug can be made. By repeating this process persons accustomed to a moderate use of sleeping pills can easily free themselves from a habit which might otherwise lead to a dangerous addiction.

be seen whether modern man is equally wise when he chooses defenses against his fears and worries.

The Stimulation in Struggle

There is ample evidence that progress upward from the lower animals to man was not made under conditions of ease, comfort, and security. In fact, students of evolution have found that when any species became so well adapted to its environment that struggle for existence was no longer necessary, its evolutionary progress ceased. It might live on for thousands or millions of years, but it never rose any higher in the scale of life, never increased the variety of its activities or the scope of its awareness. It may be, as Lecomte du Nouy has suggested in his book *Human Destiny,* that man is passing from the realm of bodily evolution into a mental and spiritual phase. If so, we should regard our internal, intangible difficulties simply as the price of further progress, as the spur to becoming more mentally alive.

History shows that tensions, apprehensions, and fears have often been stimulants to the finest and highest attainments of man. And if it is pleasure we are seeking, there is no greater source of joy in life than the discovery of effective solutions for difficult problems. When we begin to grapple with our problems and to gain glimpses of feasible solutions we will find that the worry has evaporated and that the exhilaration of victory has taken its place. But we forfeit both the mental pleasure of victory and the material rewards of constructive thinking when we meet our problems by doping our brains with tranquilizers. Someone has called our time "the age of anxiety *about* anxiety," and that is just the trouble. By turning anxiety back upon itself we make it hopeless. But anxiety directed against the causes that produced it becomes the means to progress, growth, and the most satisfying pleasures of life.

18. The mystery of
our sleep center

European Observations

It is well known that centers have been located in the brain for various functions or conditions of the body, such as breathing, circulation, and body temperature. Since sleep is one of the most important means of maintaining the body's efficiency, it seems reasonable to expect that a center would be found in the brain for its regulation.

More than fifty years ago a Viennese ophthalmologist, Ludwig Mauthner, treating the eyes of patients during an epidemic of sleeping sickness, noticed that troubles in the eye muscles and symptoms of sleeping sickness often occurred together, and from this he concluded that the eye muscles and sleep are both controlled by the same part of the brain, the bottom central part called the hypothalamus.

About twenty-five years later another Viennese physician, von Economo, during another epidemic of sleeping sickness, observed that in many of his patients an early symptom of the disease was not sleep, but absence of sleep, continued wakefulness, though when the disease had progressed further these patients fell into the continuing lethargy which is characteristic of the disease. He interpreted this to mean that there is a sleep center and also a wakefulness center in the brain, and that when the disease damages the sleep center first the patient cannot sleep, though as the disease spreads and reaches the wakefulness center he sleeps almost continuously.

More recently W. R. Hess in Switzerland, a 1949 Nobel Prize winner, has reported that by electrical stimulation of certain points in the brain of cats he was able to produce a condition with all the characteristics of natural sleep. Other experimenters, unfortunately, have been unable to duplicate Hess's results, so doubts as to their validity have arisen. But Hess's reports are in great detail and show evidence of exacting care, so it seems unlikely that he was mistaken in his observance of his results.

In America our experimenters have been reluctant to accept the existence of a sleep center, though most of them regard the existence of a wakefulness center as clearly established. Practically all agree that there is in the rear part of the hypothalamus a "sympathetic" center which is capable of stimulating various activities, while in the forward part of the hypothalamus there is a "parasympathetic" center which is able to inhibit or depress these same activities. With this much agreed, it seems highly probable that the forward part of the hypothalamus does in fact contain the sleep center proposed by von Economo and that the rear part contains also his wakefulness center, and that he was right in concluding that when disease damaged the forward part, the rear part would be left without control and so would produce the continued wakefulness which he originally observed.

After an exhaustive summary of the various ideas that have been advanced regarding the sleep center, Dr. Nathaniel Kleitman in *Sleep and Wakefulness* comes to the conclusion that the evidence available at the time he wrote was not sufficient to establish the existence of a part of the brain that could properly be called a sleep center. All the recognized features of sleep, he decided, could be satisfactorily accounted for as due to a decrease in the activity of the wakefulness center. This center he believes is kept active by nerve impulses coming from the various sense organs, such as sight and hearing and reports of muscular activity. What part the higher centers of the brain, in what is called the cortex, may play in keeping the wakefulness center active he says has not yet been determined. Sleep comes, he holds, with the reduction of the activity of the wakefulness center, and the chief factor in bringing this about is relaxation of the muscles, with the eye muscles playing a very important part.

Experiments made in Holland since Dr. Kleitman's book was published seem to the present writer, at least, to tip the balance strongly in favor of the existence of a sleep center which brings sleep by reducing or inhibiting the activity of the wakefulness center. Inhibition of activity of one nerve center by another is not a new or strange idea, but is a well-recognized feature of the activity of the nervous system. The action of the heart, for example, is regulated by two types of nerves, one to stimulate its activity, the other to reduce it, so that between the two it is controlled to meet the body's needs. There is no physiological reason why sleep should not be regulated in a similar way.

Experiments on Rats

In an effort to clear up some of the vague assumptions and inadequately based assertions which are so prevalent in discussions of the sleep center, W. J. H. Nauta, of the University of Utrecht, carried out experiments on rats which he described in the Journal of Neurophysiology for July, 1946. Instead of attempting to stimulate or destroy the nerve centers under study, Nauta used the method of isolating them by cutting the nerve fibers by which impulses from these centers are sent out to other nerve centers. This enabled him to determine what effects were caused by the impulses they send out. More than a hundred rats were used, and records kept of the effect produced in each rat by an exactly controlled cut which had been made in its brain. After allowing time for full observation the brain was removed and examined to verify the location of the cut. All cuts were made in the hypothalamus, as other experimenters had already shown that control of sleep and wakefulness is located in this part of the brain.

The results may be briefly stated as follows: When cuts were made near the front end of the hypothalamus, isolating the part where von Economo and Hess had placed the sleep center and where others had placed the parasympathetic center, the rats could not sleep. Instead of sleeping ten times a day, for a total of fourteen hours, as rats normally do, they remained continuously awake. When cuts were placed near the back part of the hypothalamus, just forward of the location commonly assigned to the wakefulness center or the sympathetic center, apparently severing fibers which might carry waking impulses forward and upward to the cortex, the rats were never awake but slept continuously. When both centers were isolated at the same time the effect was exactly the same as if only the wakefulness center alone was isolated, indicating that the sleep center did not affect the cortex directly and independently but only indirectly through inhibitions of the action of the wakefulness center.

This agrees with the conclusion of the American physiologist Ranson and his associates that sleep depends upon reduction of the waking center's activity. Ranson, however, believes that this reduction is caused, not by a sleep center, but simply by a lessening of nerve impulses which come to the waking center from various parts of the body. Since rats with the wakefulness center isolated could still be awakened by strong nerve impulses through the senses, Nauta believes that the wakefulness center merely heightens the sensitiveness of the cortex and maintains it in a condition of readiness to receive messages from the senses. Without the wakefulness center the rats, after being awakened by strong stimulation through the senses, could not maintain wakefulness, but quickly fell back into sleep. Ranson found this to be true also in monkeys, after electrical destruction of the wakefulness center.

Nauta's findings regarding the existence of a sleep center gain support through their similarity to recent findings at Harvard in experiments on the centers of hunger and satiety, which also are located in the hypothalamus. In these experiments Dr. Mayer and his colleagues discovered a drug which selectively destroyed the satiety center. Normal mice eat only until the body's needs are met. Mice with the satiety center destroyed ate continuously, increasing their weight to three or four times the normal weight. Animals with the hunger center destroyed refused to eat. These experimenters were able to determine that rapid utilization of blood sugar, denoting an abundant supply, is the condition which stimulates the satiety center and causes it to inhibit the hunger center.

It is to be hoped that these experimenters or others soon may be able to demonstrate conclusively just what the physiological conditions are that stimulate the sleep center and cause it to inhibit the wakefulness center, thus bringing sleep. Dr. Kety's experiments (Chapter One) would lead us to expect that an increase of carbon dioxide in the blood will be one of the necessary conditions.

Summary: Sleep Center or Wakefulness Center or Both, Sleep Still Takes Over If You Control Breathing

The question is now, What bearing do these various ideas of the sleep center have on our procedures for producing sleep—do they support them, or do they question them, or do they call for changes? Since our procedures depend principally on the effect of carbon dioxide, we will limit our discussion to that, and omit relaxation, eye position, and mental preoccupation. While these are important parts of the procedures, they include many details, and in some respects are based only on theory. We have, however, a well-established factual basis for judging the probable effects of carbon dioxide on the centers, whether they be sleep or wakefulness, or both. Since there is little evidence that we have a center which produces sleep by direct action on the cortex, we will not discuss that possibility.

Assuming that we have only a wakefulness center, how will an increase of carbon dioxide in the blood probably affect it? There is no basis for supposing that the effect would be different from the effect carbon dioxide has on the nervous system in general, that is, a depressant effect. So if we accept the position of Kleitman, Ranson, and others that a reduction in the activity of the wakefulness center is the determining condition of sleep, then depression of this center is the most direct possible means of bringing sleep, and our procedures are ideally adapted to meet this requirement.

If on the other hand we accept the observations of von Economo and the experiments of Nauta as indicating that there is a special sleep center which brings sleep by inhibiting the wakefulness center, there are two possible effects that an increase of carbon dioxide in the blood might produce. First, it might reduce the activity of both the sleep center and the wakefulness center. Even if this stopped the action of the sleep center completely we would still have the quieting effects on the wakefulness center, and this is the same situation we had when we assumed that we do not have a sleep center, and as we saw, this is a situation to which our procedures are well suited.

The second possible effect when we assume that we have both centers is that carbon dioxide might affect the sleep center in the same way that it does the respiratory center, that is, it might act as a stimulant, reversing its usual effect of depression. If this should prove to be the case, then our procedures could be expected to be doubly effective, both stimulating the sleep center and depressing the wakefulness center. A strong suggestion that this is actually the case comes from the fact that sleep when it is induced by controlled breathing most frequently comes suddenly with no preceding feeling of drowsiness or awareness that sleep is approaching. If sleep comes from a gradual decrease of nerve impulses that reach the wakefulness center, then we might expect its approach ordinarily to be gradual and to permit the feeling of increasing drowsiness. It seems probable that the voluntary increase of carbon dioxide in the blood arouses the sleep center and causes it to act on the wakefulness center as brakes act on a car. The car will stop gradually if the gas is cut off or the clutch released. But it will stop much more quickly if the brakes also are applied at the same time.

This sudden coming of sleep has been hard to explain on the basis of some of the current theories of sleep. Its frequent occurrence under the influence of our breathing exercises would seem to give support to the belief that we have both sleep and wakefulness centers, and that it is the stimulation of the sleep center by a voluntary increase of carbon dioxide in the blood that causes the sudden onset of sleep. However, in evaluating our procedures for bringing sleep, it is to be noted that they are in no way dependent on any particular theory regarding sleep or the sleep center. They depend first upon the practical proof of successful use, and second on a firm basis of well-known and fully recognized physiological processes. But it is interesting to find that they are also in full harmony with each of the tenable theories regarding the sleep center.

19. To sleep–to dream–
and what your dreams
can tell you

Dreams Are Normal

Dreams, so far as can be determined, are a perfectly normal type of mental activity which occurs during sleep, or more exactly, during partial sleep. It is clear from the illogical and unreasoned form of dream thoughts that the critical and discriminatory faculties of the mind are less active during their formation. Physiologists now generally agree that the thought faculties of the brain do not all become active at the same time when we awake, or cease activity at the same time when we are going to sleep. Activity of the higher centers of the brain, those which form critical judgments, disappears first and reappears last. Consequently in the interim period the more primitive thought faculties, such as memory and imagination, are able to carry on their activities without the controlling supervision or direction of the higher faculties.

As an inference from these facts the belief has long been held among physiologists and psychologists that dreams occur only or principally during these periods of partial sleep. It remained, however, for Dr. Nathaniel Kleitman, perhaps our most outstanding authority on sleep, and his associates at the University of Chicago, to devise scientific experiments for testing this belief. Having noticed intervals of eye movements during what appeared to be light sleep he suspected that they were associated with the formation of mental pictures in dreams.

Using an electroencephalograph for recording brain waves along with delicate electrical instruments for recording eye movements, Dr. Kleitman demonstrated that the eye movements did actually occur only during light or partial sleep as shown by the electroencephalograph. To test the occurrence of dreams, he waked his subjects during and after periods of eye movements. If awakened during or within fifteen minutes after a period of eye movements they were almost always able to recall the dream. Awakened at other times they seldom had any recollection of dreaming. A still more direct connection with the dream was found in the direction of the eye movements. If the dream involved climbing there were eye movements up and down. If the dream movements were on a horizontal plane the eye movements were from side to side. This is exactly the response that the eyes make to the formation of mental images when one is awake with the eyes closed.

Dr. Kleitman's experiments leave little room for doubt that dreams are produced by the brain while only part of its faculties are active. We are all aware from the character of our own dreams that they commonly show a lack of some of the most essential elements of normal waking thought. The statement, "He is not all there," which we sometimes apply colloquially to a mentally deficient person would seem to be quite literally true of all of us when we are dreaming. The critical and discriminating parts of our minds are less active, and their failure to take part in the dream thought makes possible the inclusion of the bizarre and incongruous elements which are so characteristic of dreams.

Current Thought on Dreams

It is necessary at this point to discuss in some detail the current scientific thought pertaining to the nature and meaning of dreams. Many half-truths and misconceptions are widely held in regard to dreams, and these ill-founded beliefs are likely to cause unnecessary anxiety and worry. In order to remove this disturbance of successful and restful sleep, we will examine some of the current concepts.

Dr. Kleitman's findings have established a factual physiological point of departure which must now be taken into consideration in all study and discussion of the mental activities that reach consciousness in our dreams. The bizarre character of dreams which at times may have seemed disturbing we can understand now as due to the absence of the discriminating activities of the mind, which is a characteristic of the state of partial sleep in which dreams occur. A further characteristic of the state of partial sleep is the absence of much of the usual protective covering which our minds maintain while we are normally alert in full wakefulness. And it is due to the absence of this protective covering that dreams often disclose features of the inner workings of our minds which otherwise may be hidden even from ourselves.

Very little progress had been made in penetrating this protective covering or in understanding the meaning of dreams until Doctor Sigmund Freud and his associates in Vienna began to use suggestions which they found in the dreams of their patients as aids in understanding both normal and abnormal mental functioning. Freud became convinced that dreams arose in a sleeper's mind as wish-fulfillments, the hallucinations of sleep being utilized by the dreamer for the attainment of objectives which due to the hindrance of various obstacles, he had not been able to attain while awake. The dream, by attaining the wish-fulfillment, permits the dreamer to go on sleeping. In applying this wish-fulfillment theory Freud developed his theory of three layers of mental activity, the conscious, the pre-conscious, and the unconscious, and introduced the idea of a censorship by the preconscious mind which permitted objectionable wishes to appear in a dream only in disguised form. To penetrate the disguises appearing in dreams and to find the wishes which they concealed Freud developed his now widely accepted system of dream interpretation.

Freud's work compelled the scientific world to recognize that there is much more to the human mind than appears on the surface.

To learn just what this more is many studies are underway at the present time, ranging from those of Grantly Dick Read on the electrical phenomena of the brain to those of Dr. J. B. Rhine on extrasensory perception. Since we even now have so little positive knowledge in this field, the only prudent course is to recognize our limitations and not to accept as established facts what are necessarily only inferences and theories.

Causes of Dreams

In the field of dream interpretation Freud's important contribution was his insistence that dreams do not arise without causes, and his location of these causes in what he designated as the unconscious and preconscious mind, parts of the mind which do not immediately report their activities to consciousness. As Dr. Sandor Rado of Columbia University is careful to remind us, when we come to study the unconscious activities of the mind, only the effects and derivatives of these activities can be observed. The activities themselves we cannot observe but can only infer. Freud's critics have pointed out that in some instances his inferences as to the nature of unconscious activities are without what these critics consider sufficient factual support, and consequently they regard the validity of his dream interpretations based on such inferred activities as open to question.

As a pioneer in the study of the non-reporting activities of the mind, Freud's work brought him great prominence among the students of mental activities. As a neurologist, Freud might naturally have been expected to approach the study of mental disease on a physiological basis. It seems likely that he adopted the introspective approach, utilizing the dreams of his patients as a basis for diagnosis and treatment, because the physical sciences had not then reached the point where they could be utilized for the exploration of mental processes. Freud himself did not consider his psychological treatment of mental ills as the ultimate solutions. In his book *Outline of Psychoanalysis,* Freud indicated his belief that the solution of mental ills might eventually come through chemistry, that is, through physiological chemistry, specifi-cally the chemistry of brain functions, a possibility that is now being diligently investigated in many laboratories.

Two methods for the interpretation of dreams have come to us from Eastern tradition, the recognition of symbols and the transla-tion of a cypher. The first of these methods is illustrated by the Biblical account of Pharaoh's dream in which seven fat kine represented seven fruitful years while seven lean kine represented seven years of famine. The kine are here used as symbols, and the interpretation is what is known as symbolic interpretation. Suc-cessful interpretation necessarily depends, as it did in this case, upon the interpreter's acuteness in perceiving the significance of the symbols.

The cypher method of dream interpretation depends upon the assignment of meanings to certain words that are apt to occur in dreams, these words forming a cypher or code which the interpreter uses in his interpretations. Interpretations made in this way are so plainly based on guesswork that they are not often found in present-day dream books, though the author purchased one book in his study of dreams which is made up like a dictionary or encyclopedia of an alphabetical list of words, each with a group of meanings some one of which the word is supposed to have when it occurs in a dream. The author of that book had taken care to have these meanings variable and flexible enough so that it is usually possible to choose from them a superficial but fairly plausible interpretation of most ordinary dreams. One is more likely to find in dream books a combination of the cypher method with the symbol method, in which more or less standardized mean-ings are given to certain words while meanings are assigned to other words on a supposed symbolic basis.

Freud's method of interpreting dreams discards arbitrarily as-signed meanings for dream symbols and endeavors to ascertain what ideas are associated with the dream images in the dreamer's own mind, and with these as a basis tries through the interpreter's knowledge of dream processes to construct a valid interpretation of the dream. However, Freud does list a number of dream elements as usually having a certain significance, and these have been seized on by the popular dream interpreters as lending support to their systems. Even some of Freud's professed followers have greatly extended his list of dream elements with probable symbolic meanings and may thus have unwittingly encouraged in some therapists neglect of the study of the dreamer's individual mental associations and background.

Most of the popular dream interpreters of today tend to develop their own code systems and to depend largely on their own keys for interpretations. Few of them have opportunity, time, or facilities for discovering the background and mental associations of the dreamer, which Freud emphasized as necessary for valid interpretations. Scientific students of dreams regard most popular interpretations of dreams as being in a class with astrology and palmistry.

Clues to Contents

The only kind of dream interpretation now accepted as valid by competent authorities is that used by physicians who have been trained as psychoanalysts. Being specialists in mental processes they make use of various means of probing into the unconscious activities of the mind, and one of these means is the analysis of dreams. When dreams are available they may give clues to contents and activities of the mind which do not come into consciousness under ordinary waking conditions.

Authorities now quite generally accept the fact that our minds contain much material that we are not conscious of and that they carry on various activities that we are not aware of. The unconscious mind is regarded as a sort of storehouse of our hopes, desires, purposes, aspirations, fears, frustrations and anxieties, and there can be little question that these underlying emotions have much to do with our prejudices, beliefs, preferences, attitudes, decisions, and even our actions. In the hands of a competent interpreter, dreams can often give indications of the nature and origin of this submerged material and its probable influence not only on dreams but also on the dreamer's waking thoughts and actions. The psychoanalyst finds in dreams clues that may indicate the causes of mental irregularities and suggest procedures for their correction. Psychologists also in their study of the deeper workings of the normal mind sometimes find help in the analysis of dreams. But only in rare cases are psychoanalysts or psychologists willing to base their conclusions on dreams alone. The indications they find in dreams must be combined and coordinated with information from other available sources, checked and verified by these other findings.

Because dreams are very complex in their make-up, and the processes by which they are formed are as yet only partially understood, even the best trained specialist often has difficulty in drawing indubitable inferences from them. But the chances are not very good of even a well trained specialist finding useful guidance in his personal affairs by attempting himself to interpret all of his own dreams. Interpretations by unqualified practitioners are even less likely to be useful.

A dream often appears to have a simple and natural origin in a chance grouping of past events or impressions. These materials, called by Freud the manifest content of the dream, are often brought together in the dream by a similarity or association of the most trivial or insignificant nature. In the examination of this manifest content of a dream, it is important to remember that while waking thought consists largely of ideas, relationships, and qualifications, dreams are made up almost entirely of pictures. Ideas which in waking thought are qualified by words like *if, because, though, perhaps,* etc., will appear in a dream as accomplished facts without qualifications.

In examining the manifest content of normal dreams the following kinds of dream materials are those which will be found most frequently.

(a) Events of the previous day, or of the days immediately

preceding. Often these are events which in their actual occurrence were of little or no importance.

(b) Events which made an unusually deep impression on the mind, whether recently or at a more remote time.

(c) Events of childhood, often those which had apparently been forgotten and could not have been recalled to memory when awake.

(d) Physical sensations occurring during sleep, such as cold, pressure, or any bodily discomfort. These sensations are often much exaggerated in the dream, as when a slight pressure of the bedclothes causes one to dream of being crushed by a heavy weight.

(e) Hopes, wishes, desires, purposes, strivings.

(f) Fears, worries, anxieties, frustrations, or disappointments.

Materials of this last group appear in dreams both in their true character and as their opposites. The possible event which caused the fear or anxiety may be pictured as having actually occurred, though often a different but equally disturbing event is pictured. In either case the dreamer is apt to awake in a state of deep distress. But occasionally in cases of frustration and disappointment the mind seems to seek an escape or refuge by dreaming of an experience which is especially pleasant or gratifying. In such a case the dream may be recalled upon awakening with a feeling of relief and pleasure.

In the consideration of dreams it must be remembered that dreaming is simply a process in which the dreamer may be said to stand aside and observe his own thoughts without directing them. At times he may see these thoughts more vividly or more clearly than he is able to see them when he is awake. But as a rule the information that is given by these dream pictures, either to the dreamer or to an interpreter, is about the dreamer himself, what persons or events seem to be uppermost in his mind, and how he regards these persons or events. Authenticated instances in which any other kind of information has come from a dream are so rare that no one can afford to count on it in his practical affairs.

Dreams As Unfinished Business

It has long been recognized by students of dreams that they deal almost entirely with matters which were not conclusively or completely dealt with in waking thought. In other words, dreams are made up of the mind's unfinished business. This incomplete material is of three types. First is a miscellaneous group of matters with perhaps some special interest but with no great importance. They were not followed to a conclusion in waking thought because they were crowded out by things that were more important or more urgent. Combined, often upon very tenuous associations, with more or less neutral items taken from various sources, these trivial but special-interest items make up the manifest content of the great majority of dreams of normal persons.

The other two types of dream materials are unconscious hopes and fears. Both are by nature unfinished business. They often go by other names, such as wishes and worries. Freud held that a wish and an accompanying fear might both appear in the same dream, the dreamer fearing that the forbidden unconscious wish might be acted upon in spite of the dreamer's better intentions. These two groups, unconscious wishes and fears, under their various names form what Freud called the latent content of all dreams. It is this portion of the dream, i.e., the latent content, that the psychoanalyst or the skilled psychotherapist makes use of in his efforts to help an emotionally disturbed patient. By making the patient aware of his deep unconscious worries and fears or, as Freud says, "by making the unconscious conscious," the patient is enabled to reorganize his mental life, his values, and his actions so that formerly unconscious needs are now satisfied and his fears and inner conflicts are resolved.

Another interesting class of dreams comes from the scientists and inventors who have made important discoveries or inventions in their dreams. A recent and striking example of the latter is Pierre de Fonbrune, the French biologist. He was baffled in his efforts to find a sufficiently sensitive means of manipulating the micro-tools used in dissection under the microscope until he dreamed he was moving a handle which controlled the tool through compressed air. Application of this idea solved his problem, and controls of his design are now in general use. Various other dreams of this type have been well authenticated. It is to be noted that these dreams do not come at random or by mere chance. It is only after intense application to the problem and a complete mastery of its details that the dreamer's mind, being freed by sleep from outside distractions, is able to discover a relation that had escaped him in his waking thought. As Dr. R. W. Gerard has expressed it, "The unconscious work goes on only over problems that are important to the waking mind, only when the mind's possessor worries about them, only when he cares, passionately."

This type of dream probably is closely related to what we call intuition when it occurs in our waking hours. That our minds have capabilities which we do not ordinarily use is proved by the recollection of long past and supposedly forgotten events under hypnosis. Possibly all these abilities are just the first glimmerings of slowly evolving faculties in the development of a more perfect type of human being in which intuition will become a recognized branch of science, as foreshadowed by Lecomte du Noüy in his books, *Human Destiny* and *The Road to Reason*. At present all these faculties seem to belong to the twilight zone of extrasensory perception which Dr. J. B. Rhine of Duke University has been exploring. Perhaps after a few more thousands of years of scientific investigation men will gain fuller control of these faculties and be able to put them into common and definite use. But for the present, as W. Grey Walter reminds us in his book, *The Living Brain,* we have no satisfactory explanation of hypnosis, nor has the study of brain activity thrown any satisfactory light on clairvoyance, telepathy, or extrasensory perception.

Prophetic Dreams

Another interesting class of dreams is the prophetic dream. Much of the belief in the ability of dreams to foretell the future is due to the fact that most dreams which attract attention are based on hope or fear. We only fear those things which waking reason tells us are likely to occur. If our waking judgment is good, then there is certainly more than an even chance that these things will actually happen. The more certain we are that they are going to happen, the more likely we are to dream that they have happened. If we then do dream that they have happened, can we expect anything else than that in many cases the dream should come true? In a similar manner we do not hope for things unless waking reason tells us there is a fair possibility of their realization. The more sure we are of this possibility the more earnestly we work for the realization and the more likely we are to dream of the hope as an accomplished fact. If our judgment is good and many of our hopes are attained, then a large percentage of our dreams will come true. So it is easy to see that as a game of chance the gamble is heavily weighted on the side of the fulfillment of prophetic dreams of these two classes.

Very similar to the weighted probability of fulfillment in prophetic dream is the biased evidence of dreams that seem to call for a certain course of action on the part of the dreamer. Quite commonly dreams are inspired or influenced by wishes which have been purposely suppressed or discarded because to the waking mind they are clearly unwise or impracticable. The fact that they subsequently seem to work out well in a dream certainly does not add anything to their wisdom or practicability. And in attempting to evaluate the significance of such a dream a person is biased in spite of himself, being inclined to choose an interpretation in accord with his original desires. Because both in the dream itself and again in its interpretation a dreamer is apt to be led away from reality and common sense, being guided by his previously suppressed wishes rather than his considered judgment, a dreamer's interpretation of his own dreams is certainly a doubtful guide to use in planning a course of action. It is reported that Hitler dreamed the V-2 rocket could not be used successfully against England and that as a result he opposed its advocates. If he had not allowed his dream to delay its development it might have changed the course of the war. General Dwight D. Eisenhower said that if the V-2 rocket had been completed six months earlier it might well have made the Allied invasion of Europe impossible.

Unpleasant Dreams Predominate

Statistics gathered on classes of dream show unpleasant dreams about twice as numerous as pleasant dreams. When we think of it, this is to be expected. In the first place, unpleasant experiences while awake are more apt to come under the head of unfinished business, and therefore to be proper material for dreams. A pleasant experience is regarded as completed and satisfactory, but an unpleasant experience is apt to leave one dissatisfied and wanting to do something about it. This brings it up for further consideration in a dream. In the second place, counts can be made, not of all dreams, but only of such dreams as are remembered, and it is quite possible, or even likely, that unpleasant dreams make a more vivid impression on the mind and are more likely to wake the dreamer than pleasant dreams, which causes a higher percentage of unpleasant dreams to be remembered. So no one need be disturbed if he finds a majority of his dreams more or less unpleasant. The nature of dreams would lead us to expect this in any normal person's dreams. It is only when the unpleasantness becomes extreme and persistent that it calls for further attention.

Whether ordinary unexciting dreams reduce the restfulness of sleep is open to question. There is no clear proof that they do. When they seem to do so, investigation may show that the disturbance of sleep is due to other causes, the dreaming being the result of the disturbed sleep. Most persons feel that pleasant dreams do not detract from the restfulness of sleep. Recent experiments by Dr. Nathaniel Kleitman indicate that dreaming is a normal accompaniment of sleep, and any abnormality of the dream, either in its nature or in its effect, is the result of preexisting abnormal conditions of the body or of the mind. The mere fact of dreaming, it would seem, is not in itself an indication of any pathological condition.

Sleep-Walking

Sleep-walking is often classed with dreaming. There are, however, several marked differences. Dreams are experienced by all normal persons. Sleep-walking is comparatively rare. Dreams are very commonly remembered, otherwise we would know nothing of having dreamed. But the sleep-walker usually has no recollection whatever of his sleep-walking. Apparently sleep-walking results from some mental abnormality which makes it possible for a dream under certain stresses to break through its normal barriers. Instead of merely seeing and hearing the dream action, as in normal dreams, the dreamer brings his motor mechanisms into play and acts out the dream. Sleep-walkers sometimes appear to be in much the same state as a person who has been hypnotized, being very susceptible to suggestion and disposed to do whatever they are told to do. Usually it is easy to awaken a sleep-walker by merely speaking to him quietly, though care should be taken not to awaken him when he is in a position where he might fall.

Sleep-walking should not be regarded as a normal occurrence, as it sometimes indicates an illness requiring medical attention. It may result from either physiological or psychological conditions. The fact that it frequently occurs in more than one member of a family tends to support the belief that a hereditary factor is sometimes present. Feelings of anxiety and insecurity are the common psychological causes, and they account for the great majority of cases. Infections of the brain or brain injuries may be followed by sleep-walking, and it is sometimes associated with epileptic attacks. Treatment in each case must be determined by the cause.

Talking in the sleep may be regarded as a limited type of sleep-walking in which the dream is able to break through its barriers only far enough to take over control of the speech muscles. In any case of frequent sleep-walking or sleep-talking an effort should be made to remove all sources of mental stress or worry. Also attention should be given to possible physical irritations, such as late or heavy suppers, disturbing sounds, or an uncomfortable bed.

Two other manifestations which appear to be derangements of the sleep function may be mentioned in this connection. These are narcolepsy and catalepsy. Both are apt to occur in the same person. In narcolepsy the person suddenly falls asleep even when walking or standing, then wakes after a few minutes, apparently in normal condition. In catalepsy there is a temporary complete relaxation of all muscles, so that no voluntary movement is possible, not even speech or the opening of the eyes, but there is no loss of consciousness. The cause of these afflictions is not well understood, but they can be relieved or controlled by medical treament.

Summary: Dreams? Welcome!

From all these facts about dreams we may draw several conclusions that bear on the problem of sleep. First, it is normal to dream, that is, dreams are a normal accompaniment of sleep.

Secondly, dreams do not necessarily reduce the restfulness of sleep. In fact, dreams are thought to preserve sleep many times; for example, a buzzing of an alarm clock signaling that it is time to get up may result in a dream that an airplane is passing overhead and thus distort the meaning of the sound so that the dreamer is unaware that it is time to arise and so sleep may be preserved.

Thus, as we have seen, problems may be solved during sleep and the dreamer may awake relieved of a perplexing and worrisome burden. Or a happy dream may cause us to wake with a feeling of pleasure that keeps us happy all day.

So it would appear that dreams are normally a part of the restorative and revitalizing process of sleep and as such may be welcomed into our endeavor to secure restful and refreshing sleep.

Appendix A
The secret of
slow-motion breathing
to put you to sleep

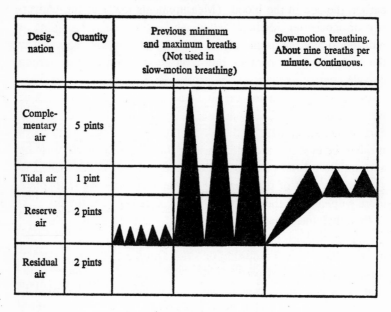

Desig-nation	Quantity	Previous minimum and maximum breaths (Not used in slow-motion breathing)	Slow-motion breathing. About nine breaths per minute. Continuous.
Comple-mentary air	5 pints		
Tidal air	1 pint		
Reserve air	2 pints		
Residual air	2 pints		

Figure 4.   Slow-Motion Breathing

Slow Down to Nine Breaths a Minute

In this supplemental type of breathing normal breaths are taken, but at only half the normal rate. When at rest we usually spend approximately the time of two heart-beats on each inhalation, and the same on each exhalation, four heart-beats for each breath. The time for each breath is now to be doubled. The rate of breathing will be about nine breaths to the minute instead of the usual eighteen. A little practice with the fingers on the pulse at the wrist will give an idea of the proper timing, allowing four beats for inhaling and four for exhaling. Care must be taken not to fill the lungs more than in ordinary quiet breathing. For this reason the breath should be taken in quite slowly, and also expelled at the same slow rate. It is this very slow rate of inhaling and exhaling that suggests the name, slow-motion breathing. It is an effective and almost effortless method of maintaining the higher content of carbon dioxide in the blood. (Measurements made at the University of Rochester Medical School show that when breathing is reduced to half the usual volume there is only a slight reduction in the body's oxygen content but a large increase in the carbon dioxide content.)

In the instructions for the first and second types of breathing we have emphasized, in addition to the maintenance of a high carbon dioxide content in the blood, the sleep-producing effects of turning the eyes upward and repeating familiar lines while forming appropriate mental pictures, these additional aids being treated as a secondary part of the breathing procedures. Now we must place more emphasis on these secondary or supplemental features.

If wakefulness has persisted through the first two types of breathing, with no pain or other physical condition to account for it, and there is no unusual outside disturbance, the persistent wakefulness is almost certainly due to a state of high mental tension. This will show itself through the wandering of the mind to disturbing thoughts which drive away sleep. In such a case there is evidently need for a stronger control of the thoughts. Fortunately the auxiliary features of our breathing procedures make it possible through their further development to gain this strong control.

Why Count Sheep?

One of these auxiliary features is potentially so effective that even in the crude form in which it has been used it has long enjoyed by far the greatest popularity of all sleep-producing devices. Everyone has heard of it, and probably most of us have used it at times, in the popular form which it has taken, the counting of sheep. The idea of wooing sleep by mentally counting sheep is based on a perfectly sound psychological principle. It is this sound basic principle that accounts for the popularity and persistence of this traditional practice. Strangely, though, it seems that no systematic effort has ever been made to find out what this basic principle is, or whether the practice is purely a superstition, without any sound basis in fact.

The psychological principle underlying sheep-counting can best be understood by thinking of the action of the mind as being similar to the action of the eye. The most sensitive part of the retina of the eye can be directed to only one object at a time, and any object that is to be seen distinctly must be held in steady focus on this part of the retina. The higher centers of the brain are like the center of the retina. They can give discriminating attention to only one thing at a time. The building of a new and definite imaginary picture in "the mind's eye" requires this exclusive discriminating attention. While the mind is occupied in forming the picture it cannot carry on another connected and continuous line of thought. Since this is true, it is possible for anyone, by requiring his mind to build a continuing series of new and different pictures to completely shut out any other line of active thought. It is our purpose now in this supplemental type of the breathing procedures to indicate means by which the full potential effectiveness of the psychological principle underlying sheep-counting can be utilized.

Counting sheep will sometimes bring sleep, especially if it is used only occasionally, or when there is only a slight tendency to wakefulness. But if it is used often, or when wakefulness is persistent, it is apt to fail. There are two definite reasons for these failures. The first is that the mental pictures constructed are all alike, so that forming them soon becomes an automatic process. Any automatic process can be carried on without requiring attention from the higher centers of the brain. So the monotonous sheep pictures, having become automatic after a little use, no longer monopolize the higher thought centers, which are then free to turn to other lines of thought. Naturally they turn to the thoughts that are most exciting, and exciting thoughts exclude sleep.

The second reason why counting sheep often fails to bring sleep is that at best its effect is exerted only on the mind. But suitable body conditions are absolutely essential to sleep, and the sheep counting ignores body conditions entirely. In our procedures control of body conditions is fundamental, including quieting of the nerves, relaxation of the muscles, moderate fatigue, and a resting position of the eyes. These are the basic factors, while other factors are brought in as auxiliaries.

Count Numbers

The first thing we must do in order to make effective use of this sheep-counting principle is to discard the sheep. As noted above, sheep pictures are too much alike. What we must have is a series of pictures that are so distinctly varied and unconventional that they compel the brain's discriminating thought centers to give them continuous attention. In addition it is important that these pictures should form a natural sequence, leading the thought from one picture to another with as little opportunity as possible for a break in the process. Furthermore, for our purpose, these pictures must be neutral and unexciting, so that they do not interfere with the coming of drowsiness. What can we use in place of the sheep that will satisfactorily meet these requirements?

The search for an answer to this question required much experimenting with many and various devices. Finally a special type of abstract counting, not associated with sheep or any other specific objects, was developed which fully met the specified requirements. It may be conveniently described as word-picture counting. Instead of imagining a series of objects, or the sounds of spoken numbers, or the forms of figures, the mind is required in this type of counting to picture the numbers as printed words spelled out in type. Even the customary spelling of the number words has been discarded, and an approximation of phonetic spelling is used instead. This change of spelling will be found a decided help in compelling the mind's close attention while forming mental pictures of the number words, which are, of course, all different. The usual sequence of the numbers supplies the desired unbroken lead from one picture to the next. And, meeting the third requirement, numbers, when they are not associated with objects, are completely neutral and unexciting. The basic numbers in this word-picture counting are: WUN, TOO, THREE, FOAR, FYV, SIX, SEVN, AYT, NYN, TEN, LEVN, TWELV.

To keep this word-picture counting in unison with the slow-motion breathing, it is necessary to lengthen out the number words to correspond with the extra long breaths. This can best be accomplished by imagining a repetition of the final letter of each number word, so that SIX becomes SIX-X-X-X, SEVN becomes SEVN-N-N-N, AYT becomes AYT-T-T-T, etc.

In order that each slow-motion count may be easily divided between inhaling and exhaling, all counts have been made to consist of either two or four syllables. Up to twelve the word *and* has been added to the name of each number to form the second syllable. In the numbers thirteen to nineteen the usual *teen* syllable has been used as the second part of the number word. Twenty, thirty, etc., becomes TWEN-TEE, THIR-TEE, etc. Above twenty the first ten numbers followed by *and* are used before the words for twenty, thirty, etc., giving WUN-AND TWEN-TEE, TOO-AND TWEN-TEE, etc.

A more soothing effect is obtained when reading these word-picture numbers as the mind projects them in their overhead position if the eyes move rhythmically, first from left to right, then from right to left, in time with the movements of inhaling and exhaling. To secure this swinging movement of the eyes the first part of each number has been made to read in the customary way from left to right, but the order of the letters in the second part of each number is reversed, and reads from right to left, that is, the letters of the second part of each number are printed in reverse order, with the first letter at the right and the last letter at the left. This arrangement avoids the sudden jerk which the eyes ordinarily make in skipping back to the left to begin the next line, for the eyes make the same movements with these imaginary numbers as in reading actual printed numbers. This left-handed reading may seem awkward at first, but the numbers are short, and with a little practice it becomes easy. And the swinging movement of the eyes which it brings is well worthwhile.

These fully detailed explanations and instructions for the word-picture counting have been given for two reasons. The first is that when properly understood and carried out this counting can give a degree of thought control that is not equalled by any other practicable device. And thought control is absolutely essential if wakefulness caused primarily by mental tension is to be overcome by our procedures. In taking sleeping pills thought control is secured by the stupefying effects of the drugs on the thought centers of the brain. But in our procedures, while the voluntary increase of carbon dioxide in the blood exerts a very definite quieting effect on the thought centers, it does not put them out of commission. Consequently in cases of high mental tension it must be supplemented by carefully chosen procedures which will bring to bear a potent psychological control. This control we get through the word-picture counting.

The second reason for full explanation of this procedure is that a full understanding of both the *how* and the *why* of it will make it much easier to learn, to remember, and to use. At first glance it may appear complicated and difficult, but once the twelve short basic number-words are learned, and the method of their combination as explained above has been grasped, the practical use of the numbers will be found surprisingly simple and easy. It presents only enough difficulty to make sure of holding the attention. Little study will be required to learn the special forms of the numbers, which are shown in full of the following page. A little preliminary practice with the eyes shut, imagining these numbers in the mind and accompanying them with the slow-motion breathing, will make them familiar.

Word-picture Numbers

To be used in unison with slow-motion breathing.

WUN   TOO   THREE   FOAR   FYV   SIX

SEVN   AYT   NYN   TEN   LEVN   TWELV

The spelling of the twelve numbers above should be made perfectly familiar before any attempt is made to use them in the word-picture counting. In learning them, the names are not merely pronounced. The eyes are to be closed and each word made to appear before the mind's eye, clearly spelled out in capital letters, just as it appears on this page. Only the numbers from one to forty are spelled out, but the count can be extended as needed, or repeated.

WUN-N-N-N D-D-D-DNA	THIR-R-R-R N-N-N-NEET	WUN-AND-D-D E-E-EET-NEWT	WUN-AND-D-D E-E-EET-RIHT
TOO-O-O-O D-D-D-DNA	FOAR-R-R-R N-N-N-NEET	TOO-AND-D-D E-E-EET-NEWT	TOO-AND-D-D E-E-EET-RIHT
THREE-E-E-E D-D-D-DNA	FIF-F-F-F N-N-N-NEET	THREE-AND-D-D E-E-EET-NEWT	THREE-AND-D-D E-E-EET-RIHT
FOAR-R-R-R D-D-D-DNA	SIX-X-X-X N-N-N-NEET	FOAR-AND-D-D E-E-EET-NEWT	FOAR-AND-D-D E-E-EET-RIHT
FYV-V-V-V D-D-D-DNA	SEVN-N-N-N N-N-N-NEET	FYV-AND-D-D E-E-EET-NEWT	FYV-AND-D-D E-E-EET-RIHT
SIX-X-X-X D-D-D-DNA	AYT-T-T-T N-N-N-NEET	SIX-AND-D-D E-E-EET-NEWT	SIX-AND-D-D E-E-EET-RIHT
SEVN-N-N-N D-D-D-DNA	NYN-N-N-N N-N-N-NEET	SEVN-AND-D-D E-E-EET-NEWT	SEVN-AND-D-D E-E-EET-RIHT
AYT-T-T-T D-D-D-DNA	TWEN-N-N-N E-E-E-EET	AYT-AND-D-D E-E-EET-NEWT	AYT-AND-D-D E-E-EET-RIHT

| NYN-N-N-N | NYN-AND-D-D | NYN-AND-D-D |
| D-D-D-DNA | E-E-EET-NEWT | E-E-EET-RIHT |

| TEN-N-N-N | TEN-AND-D-D | TEN-AND-D-D |
| D-D-D-DNA | E-E-EET-NEWT | E-E-EET-RIHT |

LEVN-N-N-N
D-D-D-DNA

TWELV-V-V-V
D-D-D-DNA

The fact that these imaginary word-picture numbers can easily be projected overhead gives them a great additional advantage over the counting of sheep. Sheep we naturally think of as being on the ground, and this keeps our eyes in the horizontal position. But by imagining these word-picture numbers as appearing on the ceiling, or in any position overhead, we can cause our eyes to turn upward during the word-picture counting and the accompanying slow-motion breathing. In this way we enlist a third natural aid to sleep. Different theories have been offered to explain why turning the eyes upward should be an aid in bringing sleep. These were discussed fully in Chapter Thirteen. That turning the eyes upward is a definite aid to sleep is no longer open to question.

In carrying out the word-picture counting the count may sometimes be lost. This may occur from either of two causes. (1) The mind may drop the word-picture counting and go off on some other line of thought. This indicates that the word-pictures were not being held distinctly and persistently before the mind's eye. The remedy is to give closer attention to these pictures. (2) Consciousness may be lost for just an instant. This is a favorable sign and means that sleep is approaching. Whatever may cause the interruption, the counting should start again promptly, beginning where it was dropped as nearly as can be remembered. The exact point of restarting is of no importance.

The breathing, too, may sometimes be interrupted by a sudden, sharp inhalation. This is due to involuntary nerve action and gives relief from the fatigue of continued restraint in the slow-motion

breathing. It may indicate that the slow breaths have been somewhat more shallow than necessary, but it does not require a corrective change in the breathing. After exhaling the air taken in by
this sharp inhalation, the counting and slow breathing should be
resumed and carried on as before.

The word-picture numbers listed have been carried only up to
forty. In practice it will not often be possible to follow them this
far before they are interrupted by sleep. Only occasionally can one
continue them to this point and still be awake. In such a case the
same scheme of counting can easily be carried on as far as one
hundred if desired.

Time Required

The reader may wonder how much time these various breathing
procedures will take. The first type of breathing usually continues
three to five minutes, the second type five to ten minutes, and the
supplemental type, slow-motion breathing, three to five minutes, a
total of from eight to twenty minutes. These are averages. Frequently sleep comes in the first ten minutes. In stubborn cases each
type of breathing may be extended almost indefinitely. In any case
the bringing of natural sleep is abundantly worth the time. Even if
sleep should fail to come after persistent use of the breathing
procedures, it is infinitely better to have spent the time in these calm,
constructive, and relaxing exercises than to have spent it in nervous
tossing and fretful worring, which in most cases is the insomniac's
customary procedure.

If one is still awake after faithfully carrying out instructions for
all types of breathing, there is nothing to prevent him from starting
the whole process over again. Some of the effects of the first trial
will remain, especially the fatigue and relaxation, and a second
trial can start with this advantage. Since the procedures are all perfectly wholesome, there is no reason why one should not continue
into a second and even a third trial if necessary.

But before starting a second trial it is best to have a short rest
period in which all effort is stopped, the breathing becoming auto-

matic and unconscious and the thoughts being allowed to follow any pleasant and undisturbing line that suggests itself. It often happens that this stopping of effort permits sleep to follow almost immediately.

If sleep does not come within a few minutes, or if disturbing thoughts continue to intrude themselves, then a new start should be made, beginning with the first type of breathing and going on from there with a firm determination to adhere even more closely than before to the procedures as they are outlined in the instructions.

Breaths Not Pain-Killers

As stated previously, these breathing procedures are not effective as pain killers, and therefore cannot be substituted for proper treatment of the disease which caused the pain. Often, however, the wakefulness which accompanies disease is due, not to pain, but to worry over the possible consequences of the disease. In such cases these procedures are just as appropriate and just as effective as in overcoming worry due to other causes. Their conveniences and adaptability and the absence of any hangover effect make them especially gratifying to the invalid.

In the case of a few diseases, while there is no pain, there is nevertheless a persistent wakefulness. Among these are diseases of the thyroid gland, the prostate gland, and the liver, as well as high blood pressure, anemia, certain defects of the eyes, and the after effects of sleeping sickness. Some mental disorders are likely to be associated with persistent wakefulness. Any wakefulness which cannot be overcome by a determined trial of the procedures outlined in this book may be a symptom of disease, requiring competent medical attention.

Summary: Habit Plus Faith Equals Sleep

The various types of breathing procedures are aimed primarily to enlist the aid of increased carbon dioxide, fatigue, mental picture forming, and eye position in bringing sleep, but as one continues to use them it will be found that two additional aids are gradually building up. The first is the habit of going to sleep under the influence of these procedures—a conditioned reflex, psychologists would call it. No one knows just what the process is by which we pass from wakefulness to sleep. But we all know that we cannot bring on this change by voluntary effort, such as we would use in closing our eyes or taking a deep breath. Whatever the process of going to sleep is, it is certainly involuntary. And a well-established conditioned reflex can exert a powerful influence over any involuntary process.

The second aid that builds up is confidence that these procedures, persistently carried out, can and will bring sleep. This confidence reaches the point of what we might call faith. We confidently believe that, under reasonable conditions, sleep is now at our command. When this faith comes, one of the greatest and most stubborn obstacles to sleep, the fear of wakefulness, is gone.

Sleep induced by these breathing procedures will be found to have two characteristics that at first may seem surprising. The first is the almost complete absence of what is known as the sleep start, or more technically as "physiological hypnic myoclonias." These unpleasant sudden wakenings just after going to sleep are caused by spasmodic muscular contractions. Like all muscular contractions they occur in response to nervous impulses, and the impulses which cause these starts are now known to come from a definite location in the brain. Their suppression by the breathing procedures undoubtedly is due to the increase of carbon dioxide in the blood. Here we have clear evidence of the quieting effect of carbon dioxide on the brain and its relaxing effect upon the muscles. There is wonderful comfort in knowing when one lies down to sleep that he has the means of wholesomely reducing nervous and muscular tensions before he goes to sleep so that these sleep starts will not jerk him back into wakefulness after sleep has been won.

A second characteristic of the sleep that follows these breathing procedures is that it often comes without warning. It is quite usual for a person going to sleep to pass through a period in which he realizes that he is almost asleep, though he is still conscious. This condition is known to physiologists as the hypnagogic state. But when using the breathing procedures this state is quite likely to be absent. And after one has slept, he is apt to wake with the feeling that he has not been asleep, since he has no recollection of having gone to sleep, of waking, or of dreaming. But a look at the clock brings the realization that so much time could not pass unawares except in sleep. This experience simply means that one has slept so soundly that he has indeed been "dead to the world."

Appendix B
Why we breathe—
and what are the
effects of changes
in breathing

Results of Over-breathing

The first step in understanding the effect of voluntarily increased or decreased breathing is to realize that the effect, so far as the brain and consciousness are concerned, is just the opposite of what would naturally be expected.

The primary purpose of all breathing is to have the blood absorb oxygen from the air while both the blood and the air are passing through the lungs. In ordinary breathing the amount of air breathed in and out is unconsciously regulated to ensure that the blood receives a full load of oxygen to carry to the various parts of the body, or to use more technical terms, to ensure that the blood as it leaves the lungs is practically one hundred per cent saturated with oxygen. Since normal involuntary breathing gives practically one hundred per cent saturation, it is at once evident that breathing more than the normal amount of air will not materially increase the amount of oxygen carried by the blood.

While consciously increasing the rate of breathing does not put more oxygen into the blood, it does wash more carbon dioxide out of the blood, so that the amount of carbon dioxide in the blood when it leaves the lungs is much less than in normal breathing. But any change in the carbon dioxide content of the brain's blood supply at once affects the brain's activity. Consequently it is necessary that the amount of carbon dioxide in the brain's circulation should be held to only a slight variation, and for this control the brain has its own special provision.

When the carbon dioxide in the blood coming to the brain from the lungs falls below normal, the blood vessels of the brain contract and slow the passage of the blood, so that the carbon dioxide which is being produced in the brain accumulates in the slow-moving blood sufficiently to restore the normal amount of carbon dioxide. But while the blood is moving slowly to accumulate carbon dioxide it necessarily has more of its load of oxygen used up than it ordinarily would, and since it had no increased load to start with, its oxygen content, instead of being increased by the increased breathing, is reduced below normal. An extreme degree of over-breathing can actually reduce the oxygen supply of the brain sufficiently to cause fainting, loss of consciousness, which is simply a failure of the brain's activity. The increase of breathing which one would naturally expect to increase the brain's supply of oxygen actually results in starving it of oxygen, because the reduction of carbon dioxide contracts the brain's blood vessels and slows its circulation.

As it is easy to increase the amount of air one breathes, it is just as easy, by taking slower or shallower breaths, to reduce it. And here also the effect on the brain is just the opposite of what might be expected.

Results of Under-breathing

Since normal involuntary breathing provides a large surplus of air to guarantee full saturation of the blood with oxygen, a moderate reduction in the amount of air that is breathed causes little or no reduction in the blood's supply of oxygen. But any reduction in breathing, small or large, causes a proportional reduction in the amount of carbon dioxide washed out of the blood, so that an increased amount of carbon dioxide remains in the blood as it leaves the lungs. This increase causes dilation of the blood vessels of the brain and so increases the amount of blood flowing through the brain. This increased flow, resulting from a moderate reduction in breathing, instead of reducing the brain's supply of oxygen, actually results in making an increased amount of oxygen available to the brain. This, of course, does not mean that the brain will use more oxygen, for the brain, like other parts of the body, uses only as much oxygen as its activities require, with the blood still carrying the increased amount when it returns to the lungs.

As long as the increase or decrease of breathing is only moderate the effect is the opposite of what we would expect, that is, an increase of breathing decreases the supply of oxygen to the brain and a decrease of breathing increases the brain's oxygen supply. This paradoxical effect is abolished when the increase or decrease of breathing is carried to extremes, such as complete stopping of breathing, or long and vigorous over-breathing, for then the situation changes, and both produce the same result, that is a shortage in the oxygen supply of the brain. When breathing is greatly reduced the air reaching the lungs is not sufficient to give the blood its normal supply of oxygen to carry to the brain. When breathing is greatly increased the reduction of carbon dioxide causes the blood vessels of the brain to contract so strongly that not enough blood can pass through them to bring in the amount of oxygen which the brain needs. A sufficiently strong-willed person can carry either extreme far enough to cause fainting. Fortunately, when unconsciousness results, either from over- or from under-breathing, purposeful control of the breathing ceases, and involuntary control soon brings the oxygen supply of the brain back to normal and consciousness is restored.

Since the effectiveness of the procedures recommended in this book for the production of sleep depend to a large extent on the effects of reduced breathing, it is worthwhile to examine these procedures somewhat in detail. The first step suggested in reduction is breath-holding, complete suspension of breathing, for as long as it can be maintained without discomfort (considerably less than a minute for the average person). The reduction of the oxygen content of the blood during this time is not sufficient to affect the brain, especially since it is largely counterbalanced by the increased blood flow. Immediately following the period of breath-holding, the reduction of oxygen in the blood is almost completely overcome by the three maximum breaths which follow, so that this sequence of alternating periods of breath-holding and maximum breaths can be continued indefinitely without any perceptible lack of oxygen.

In the second type of breath control, where a series of very shallow breaths is used instead of breath-holding, the effect so far as oxygen supply is concerned is essentially the same as in the first type, since it also provides adequate oxygen. The third type of breath control, using breaths of normal size, but at a slower rate, is not noticeably different from the first two in its effect on the oxygen supply, if the depth and speed of the breaths are properly regulated. Either type of breath control may be continued as long as desired without causing any harm or even noticeable discomfort.

Our Store of Oxygen

For those who like their information in the form of figures, the effect of a period of breath-holding upon the oxygen of the blood may be stated as follows. The amount of blood circulating in a man's body is about five quarts, most commonly given as five liters. One-fourth of this, called arterial blood, is in the arteries on its way from the lungs and heart to the various parts of the body, and is carrying a full charge of oxygen, about 18 or 19 per cent. The remaining three-fourths, called venous blood, is in the slow venous circulation on its way back to the heart and lungs. It, of course, carries somewhat less oxygen, averaging about 14 per cent. Since one liter contains one thousand centimeters, calculation from the percentages given will show 225 cc. of oxygen in the arterial blood and 525 cc. in the venous blood, a total of 750 cc. A man at rest, as he would be when preparing for sleep, uses about 250 cc. of oxygen per minute, so the oxygen in his blood at the start of a period of breath-holding, if he could use it up completely, would be enough to supply his needs for three minutes. Few people can hold the breath longer than a minute, indicating that nature has given us a considerable margin for safety. The average comfortable time of breath-holding as suggested in our procedures, starting with the lungs as empty as possible, is 40 seconds, two-thirds of a minute. So it is evident that at the end of a period of breath-holding the blood still contains a good reserve of unused oxygen, approximately 583 cubic centimeters, more than the body at rest uses in two minutes.

The figures given here are based on many careful measurements and are reliable for the first period of breath-holding. But they do not hold for the second breath-holding period, because the period of maximum breaths which comes between, about a third of a minute, is not long enough to completely restore the oxygen content of all the blood to the degree of saturation which it had when the first period of breath-holding was started. Only half of the oxygen used by the body during the 40 seconds of breath-holding is restored. The other half, about 83 cubic centimeters, remains as a shortage. Also it must not be overlooked that the body has continued to use oxygen during the 20 seconds of maximum breaths. During this time another 83 cubic centimeters is used which must be added to the deficit. So at the end of the second period of breath-holding the reserve of unused oxygen in the blood will be 166 cubic centimeters less than at the end of the first breath-holding period. Instead of a reserve of 583 cubic centimeters the reserve will be only 417 cubic centimeters.

This reserve of 417 cubic centimeters of oxygen is still more than half of the original content of the blood, which was 750 cubic centimeters when breath-holding was started, so that it is still well above the one-third of saturation below which the shortage of oxygen would begin to affect the brain. But a third period of breath-holding at the same rate of depletion would reduce the blood's oxygen to the marginal reserve of 250 cubic centimeters. Since no further reduction could be tolerated, it would seem to be necessary at this point to resume continuous breathing in order to replenish the oxygen supply. In practice, however, this does not prove to be necessary, for as stated above the alternating periods of breath-holding and maximum breaths can be continued indefinitely without producing any perceptible lack of oxygen.

Here, as is often the case, our attempts to calculate what will happen in our bodies under given conditions does not prove out in practice, because the body's activities are so complex that we are almost certain to overlook some significant factors. What then have we overlooked in this calculation? Of course, if it had been possible, we should have used actual measurements instead of making calculations. But the conditions we are dealing with change so rapidly that measurements would be practically impossible, and any measurement we might make would be less reliable than our calculation. So we have followed the most dependable course open to us, that is, to calculate from the reliable measurements we had, check the results in practice, and then search our calculations to find where they slipped up.

The first slip we find was in overlooking the residual air in the lungs. This air, about two pints (1 liter, 1000 cubic centimeters) at the end of a period of maximum breathing is very rich in oxygen, containing much more than the 14 per cent usually estimated for the air in the lungs during quiet breathing. Even at 14 per cent it would contain 140 cubic centimeters of oxygen, and if even only part of this were taken up by the blood during the period of breath-holding it would go far to reduce the deficit which our calculation indicated. And the average amount of residual air is in fact considerably greater than the two pints used in our calculations. This air cannot be measured directly, and there is great variation from person to person. Even for women the average is probably greater than two pints, and for men it is much greater, possibly double. Certainly for men this larger amount of residual air, if used in our calculations, would show an oxygen supply more than ample at the end of the three periods of breath-holding. And in the case of women the amount of oxygen used is actually about twenty per cent less than the 250 cubic centimeters per minute used in our calculations, giving them also a considerable margin above our figures. In order to be on the conservative side, we used in our calculations the larger figure for oxygen use and the small figure for reserve air.

Your Oxygen Shortage Prevented

Another reason why a shortage of oxygen does not occur during successive periods of maximum breaths and breath-holding is that the amount of oxygen absorbed by the blood during each period of maximum breaths is not a fixed quantity but increases as needed to give the blood leaving the lungs a full charge of oxygen. Because of this variation any shortage of oxygen in the blood when it returns to the lungs increases the amount of oxygen which it will take up, and this increase in uptake means a decrease in the shortage.

Another factor which probably helps to reduce the oxygen deficit is the short distance which the blood has to travel to and from the brain. The brain always uses a large part of the oxygen from the blood passing through it, using just as much when at rest as when at work. Blood passing through the lungs near the end of a period of breath-holding cannot be fully recharged with oxygen. Passing on to the brain this blood must meet heavy oxygen demands, almost completely exhausting its supply. But the short distance it has to travel probably brings much of it back to the lungs in the midst of the next period of maximum breaths, when abundant oxygen is present. Having been doubly depleted, it now takes up a correspondingly large amount of oxygen, much more than the amount used in our calculations. This extra amount means just that much reduction in the deficit which our calculations showed.

A still further factor that is probably of considerable importance in this connection is the body's increasingly relaxed condition brought about by the increase of carbon dioxide in both blood and tissues as the controlled breathing progresses. One important effect of this relaxation is a reduction in the oxygen used by the body in maintaining muscle tone, so that it is actually using much less than the 250 cubic centimeters a minute on which our calculations were based.

Figures cannot be given for these different compensating factors, because they are not subject to direct measurement nor even to dependable calculation. But it is clear that taken together they are easily capable of making up the entire deficiency of oxygen indicated by our calculations. For proof that they do make it up, we can only fall back on the countless tests in actual practice that have been made of the breathing procedures. In no case has a perceptible shortage of oxygen developed.

The only point in the breath-holding procedures where a reduced supply of oxygen may be expected to play a part is in the optional procedure suggested in Chapter 6. In this special procedure continuation of the maximum breaths with no intervals of breath-holding washes carbon dioxide out of the circulating blood and compels the brain to contract its blood vessels and slow the circulation in order to make up the deficiency of carbon dioxide by retaining most of what the brain itself produces. Apparently the reason for this automatic retention of carbon dioxide is to maintain a normal acid-base balance in the brain. But if this reduction of the circulation is carried far enough it will limit the brain's supply of oxygen to the point where it is no longer able to maintain consciousness, and fainting will result. *In our procedure no one is asked to go to such an extreme, but merely to the point where oxygen reduction begins to slow the brain's activity. Then by switching quickly to breath-holding some of this slowing can be carried over and added to the quieting effect of the carbon dioxide increase which immediately results from minimum breathing. By combining two brain-slowing effects in this way sleep can often be induced very quickly.*

Another Gas We Breathe

Oxygen and carbon dioxide are not the only gases in the air that we breathe. They do not even make up the principal part of it. Most of the air is nitrogen, 79 per cent, almost four-fifths. So far as the chemical processes of the body are concerned however, the nitrogen of the air is completely inactive. As the chemists say, it is inert. It does not enter into chemical combination with other elements present in the body. This is not to say that nitrogen is not used by the body. It is used very extensively. But it can be used only when received in combination with other elements in the proteins of food. Since it is inactive in our bodies in the uncombined form in which it is found in the air, breathing more or less of it does not affect our body processes. It does, though, permeate our bodies in solution in the body fluids. Under ordinary conditions we are not conscious of its presence. The air contains also a few other gases such as helium, argon, and xenon, but these are in very minute quantities, and they are inert, taking no part in the body's chemical processes.

Compared with the nitrogen and oxygen, the amount of carbon dioxide in the air that we inhale is extremely small, only about three-hundredths of one per cent. But the body does not draw its supply from this small fraction. In sharp contrast with its dependence on the surrounding air for its supply of oxygen, the body is constantly producing carbon dioxide in quantities much larger than are required for its own needs. Another contrast with oxygen is in storage capacity. Nearly all the body's oxygen is stored in the blood, and this storage is very limited, the supply being sufficient for only a few minutes, even when the body is completely at rest. The blood serves also as a storage for carbon dioxide, principally in the combined form of sodium bicarbonate. In addition large quantities of carbon dioxide are contained in all parts of the body. While there is little room for variation in the body's oxygen supply without serious damage, large quantities of the stored carbon dioxide can be thrown off by increased breathing, or large quantities added to it by reduced breathing, without undesirable effects.

One of our breath-control procedures, the slow motion breathing, since it continues over a considerable period without variation, brings the body's content of both oxygen and carbon dioxide to a steady state and maintains this state long enough for accurate measurement. Such a measurement has been made at the University of Rochester Medical School. It shows that a reduction of half in the volume of air breathed, which is the effect of our slow motion breathing when carefully carried out, will cause a reduction in the body's oxygen content of about half a pint, one-fourth of a liter. More than twice this reduction could be made before any significant lack of oxygen would occur. This same rate of breathing, however, causes an increase in the body's content of carbon dioxide of sixteen times this amount, a total of four liters. The reduction of oxygen occurs almost entirely in the blood, as there is very little storage of oxygen in the other parts of the body. The great increase in carbon dioxide is possible because it is stored not only in the blood but in all the fluids and tissues of the body. By contrast these measurements showed that when the volume of breathing is doubled the amount of oxygen in the body, including the blood, is increased only twenty cubic centimeters, about one-fiftieth of a quart, though this doubled breathing washes out of the body and blood more than a quart and a half of carbon dioxide, seventy-five times as much as the increase of oxygen.

Summary: Benefits Reviewed

As shown by these measurements, it is very easy to increase greatly the amount of carbon dioxide in the blood by breathing just enough air to maintain the blood's supply of oxygen but not enough to carry out of the lungs as much carbon dioxide as the body is producing. The resulting increase of carbon dioxide produces its major effect in the body through a reduction in the excitability of the nerves, including the brain and other parts of the nervous system. This effect of carbon dioxide was discussed in chapter 16. A second important effect of increased carbon dioxide is dilation of the blood vessels of the skin. This was discussed in the same chapter. A third effect may properly be called secondary, since it is produced through the primary effect of reduced excitability of the nerves. It is an unconscious relaxation of the voluntary muscles. This is only slightly less important than the primary effect in bringing sleep. Nerve impulses are the great enemy of sleep, and one of the principal sources of these impulses is in the voluntary muscles when they are in a state of contraction. Even the mild, steadily maintained contraction called muscle tonus sends disturbing nerve impulses to the brain. Since tonus is maintained by unconscious reflex action, attempts to release it by conscious effort produce little if any effect. But a simple and prompt means of relaxing tonus and removing it as a hindrance to sleep is afforded by the unconscious relaxing effect of carbon dioxide. This effect was discussed in Chapter Eleven.

Appendix C
How an amazing gas
does so many things for us

The Many Uses of CO_2

Since control of the amount of carbon dioxide in the body constitutes the basis of the procedures described in this book for use
as a means of inducing sleep, the reader may be interested in some
of the other uses which this versatile gas has been made to serve.

Carbon dioxide is a basic factor in the support of all life upon
the earth. Life depends upon a constant expenditure of energy.
The source of this energy is the sun. But sunlight is not continuous.
So in order to be constantly available, this energy must be caught
and stored. Plants have the ability to take up water from the soil
through their roots and to take in carbon dioxide from the air
through their leaves. Then by means of the green chlorophyl in
their leaves they are able to combine water and carbon dioxide
in such a way as to form sugar, starch (grains), and cellulose (the
stems of plants), with the energy of sunlight stored in the mole-
cules of these food substances. In these foods both plants and
animals have a source of stored energy which can be used as it
is needed in their life processes to maintain growth and activity.
When the energy from these foods is used, the water and carbon
dioxide are released, ready to be used again in another cycle of
energy storage and use. The process by which these two free and
abundant substances are utilized to catch and store the energy of
sunlight in food substances is called photosynthesis. When scien-

tists learn how to duplicate this process in their laboratories, much of the world's food will be produced in factories, using these same two cheap raw materials, water and carbon dioxide.

Plants in taking up water from the soil take up also various minerals in solution in the water and build these minerals into their seeds and stalks. Animals eating the plants obtain the same minerals and use them in their body chemistry and body structure. One of the most important of these minerals is calcium, which is familiar to everyone as calcium oxide or calcium hydroxide, both commonly known as lime. And here again carbon dioxide plays a vital part in every animal's life, for it combines with calcium to form calcium carbonate, one of the essential materials of which bones are made. Without the strength and firmness of our bones, life as we know it would be impossible.

By a figure of speech we might say that the bones of the earth itself are made up largely of this same substance, calcium carbonate, which as it occurs in the surface of the earth is commonly known as limestone. We often hear the expression "rock-ribbed hills," and all over the earth limestone ledges can be seen projecting from the hillsides. Without these ledges and the products made from them many of our most important industries would be seriously handicapped, or would no longer exist at all.

If food and bones are important to life, what shall we say of breathing? And what is it that regulates our breathing to give us always an adequate supply of oxygen from the air? One would naturally suppose that the amount of oxygen in the blood would be the basis for the control of breathing. But tests have shown that it is not the blood's content of oxygen but its content of carbon dioxide that is the principal regulator of breathing. A special sensitiveness to carbon dioxide gives the respiratory center of the brain extremely close control of breathing. Even a slight increase of carbon dioxide in the blood causes an immediate increase in breathing until the excess above normal is carried away in the breath. Correspondingly a slight decrease of carbon dioxide in the blood brings a decrease in breathing which allows the carbon dioxide produced in the body to accumulate until the blood's content comes up again to normal. Since carbon dioxide is produced from the oxygen taken in by breathing, the regulation of breathing by the amount of carbon dioxide produced guarantees replacement of the oxygen as rapidly as it is used.

Our Acid-alkali Balance

The acid-alkali balance of the blood is just as essential to life as the blood's supply of oxygen, and here, too, carbon dioxide is the primary means of regulation. When carbon dioxide is washed out of the blood by rapid breathing, the reaction swings toward the alkaline side. When the rate of breathing is not great enough to carry carbon dioxide away as fast as it is formed in the body, the acid-alkali balance swings toward the acid side, producing what doctors call respiratory acidosis. But since any excess of carbon dioxide in the arterial blood acts as a stimulant to the respiratory center, breathing is promptly increased sufficiently to remove the excess of carbon dioxide, and the acid-alkali balance swings back to normal.

Even in the digestion of our food carbon dioxide plays an important part. Hydrochloric acid, often called muriatic acid, is necessary for the digestion of protein foods in the stomach, such as meat, eggs, and milks. This acid comes from the salt which is always present in the blood. Salt is sodium chloride, hydrochloric acid combined with sodium. In order to release the hydrochloric acid when it is needed for digestion, another acid must be substituted. The substitute acid used by the stomach for this replacement is carbonic acid, and this is produced by combining carbon dioxide and water, both of which are always available in practically unlimited quantities. Thus we see that carbon dioxide is essential, not only in the production of foods, but also in preparing them for use in the body.

Another important action of carbon dioxide in the body is its relaxing effect upon the blood vessels of muscles which are doing work. Muscular energy is produced by a chemical combination of oxygen with sugar which is carried in the blood in the form of glucose. Combination of oxygen with the carbon of glucose produces carbon dioxide. The relaxing effect of the carbon dioxide which this produces causes the small blood vessels of the muscle to enlarge, so that more blood flows through the muscle, in this way bringing increased supplies of oxygen and glucose. This locally selective process has the great advantage of bringing an extra supply of blood to just the muscle or muscles that are in need of it, without disturbing the circulation in the remainder of the body.

These are only a few of the important natural uses of carbon dioxide in the body. There are various other uses of equal or almost equal importance, not all of which are fully understood at present. In addition there are various artificial or man-made uses. Among these are several important medical uses.

As mentioned earlier, carbon dioxide was the first general anesthetic used for surgical operations in pioneer experiments on animals, when sleep was produced with carbon dioxide from the animal's own breath. Other substances with longer lasting effects were later found to be better suited for surgical anesthesia. Recently doctors in Chicago and Milwaukee began testing carbon dioxide in the treatment of mental patients. Inhalation of carbon dioxide mixtures of 30 per cent, with 70 per cent of oxygen produced a deep sleep from which patients awoke relaxed and comfortable. They were able to see their problems more normally and to face them with new courage. To test the effects of this treatment one doctor took it himself nearly a hundred times. It brought him refreshing sleep with no unpleasant after-effects.

Used in Childbirth

Another recent medical use of carbon dioxide is for the purpose of reducing the labor pains of childbirth. Though not widely adopted as yet, carbon dioxide is claimed to have many advantages over other anesthetics that are in general use. One very important advantage is that it has been found to be a help instead of a hindrance in starting the baby to breathe.

Hourly inhalations of carbon dioxide are used in the new narcosis treatment for epilepsy recently developed at the Cedars of Lebanon Hospital in Los Angeles. And in many hospitals inhalations of carbon dioxide are given to patients who are waking from sleep following surgical operations. They wake with much less discomfort, and in addition this treatment has been found to greatly reduce the occurrence of postoperative pneumonia, probably because it clears the lungs by stimulating breathing.

Dr. L. J. Meduna, of the University of Illinois, who pioneered the use of carbon dioxide in the treatment of mental patients, has recently found through experiments on animals that inhalation of carbon dioxide produces measurable effects on the secretion of hormones by the endocrine glands, including the pituitary, the adrenals, and the thyroid, the effect on the thyroid being a reduction of the secretion. When these effects can be measured and controlled a large field will almost certainly be opened for the use of carbon dioxide in medical practice.

In tests at the University of Illinois it was found that all the anesthetics in common use gradually reduce and finally reverse the normal negative electrical polarity of the surface of the brain, but carbon dioxide reduced and reversed the polarity more rapidly and more completely than any of the other anesthetics in the test. The principal reason why carbon dioxide is not used in surgical operations is that its effect does not last long enough. However, the U. S. Public Health Service has found it an ideal anesthetic for use in handling flies while short lengths of nylon thread in different colors are being glued to their bodies. The colored threads make it possible for scientists to identify different groups of flies after they have been released and so to learn the flight range, rate of dispersion, and other characteristics of these pests.

Cure for Hiccups

A quite common use of carbon dioxide by physicians is in the treatment of severe hiccups. Hiccups are caused by involuntary contractions of the muscles of the diaphragm, and the quieting and relaxing effects of carbon dioxide taken into the blood by breathing mixtures of this gas in air or oxygen, are often sufficient to stop these spasmodic contractions when other remedies have failed. A popular form of this treatment is breathing into a paper bag and so taking back into the lungs the carbon dioxide which had been thrown out in previous breaths. It is possible that other popular remedies for hiccups, such as fright or surprise, taking nine swallows of water, or an effort to drink from the far side of a cup, owe their effect partly at least to the temporary holding of the breath which they cause, thus retaining some extra carbon dioxide in the lungs.

The inhalation of five per cent carbon dioxide in oxygen has long been used in hospitals as a treatment for the purpose of dilating the arteries of the brain. Persons who suffer from hardening of the arteries and high blood pressure are liable to attacks of dizziness resulting from contraction of the brain's arteries. This reduces the blood flow and consequently the oxygen supply of the brain. Physicians are now advising such patients to ward off these attacks by carrying a paper bag and beginning to breathe into it at the first sign of dizziness. Air breathed into the bag contains a considerable amount of carbon dioxide, and five or ten deep breaths of it are usually sufficient to ward off the threatened attack.

It is not generally known, but some if not all of the famous Dionne quintuplets probably owe their lives to the skillful and timely use of carbon dioxide by Dr. Dafoe. This was the first quintuple birth in medical history in which all the babies survived. More than twenty-five years ago rescue crews of the Chicago Fire Department began using carbon dioxide for the revival of newborn babies who had failed to breathe, and since that time many lives have been saved by its use. The time-proved method of reviving the baby by blowing into its mouth undoubtedly owed its success largely to the fact that the air thus forced into the baby's lungs contained up to as much as five per cent of carbon dioxide, though the original practitioners of this method, of course, never suspected that this was a factor in reviving the baby. Mouth-to-mouth artifi-

cial respiration is now widely approved as a method of resuscitation, and it is unquestionably superior in many cases to other methods. One reason for its superiority is that it not only forces oxygen into the lungs, but also supplies carbon dioxide to stimulate the respiratory center of the brain.

Helps Asthmatics

In Germany during World War II asthmatics found that they breathed more easily while seeking refuge from Allied bombs in the Kluert caves in the Ruhr. Now many German asthmatics go there for relief. The effect is believed to be due to the high carbon dioxide content of the air in the caves, which tends to diminish the spasms of the muscle fibers in the walls of the bronchial tubes.

One of the most recent medical uses of carbon dioxide is in a treatment to relieve the symptoms of multiple sclerosis, a nerve disorder which is not yet well understood. Relief is believed to come through prevention of spasms in the small blood vessels. This is similar to the cure of hiccups by preventing spasms of the diaphragm. Since carbon dioxide is known to be an effective dilator of the blood vessels, it seems probable that the relief it gives comes through an improved blood supply to the affected nerves.

Carbon dioxide now plays an important part in the diagnosis of cancer. While the patient lies on the operating table a small portion of the suspected tumor is instantly frozen with compressed carbon dioxide gas. While frozen solid it is placed in a microtome and sliced to incredible thinness. Placing one of these almost transparent slices in a microscope the pathologist examines it and can tell immediately whether the tumor is malignant, that is, a cancer, or whether it is benign, non-cancerous. In this way the surgeon knows without delay what his procedure must be.

Carbon dioxide in the form of dry ice furnishes one of the safest and most successful treatments for the removal of warts. The wart is first pared until it is almost ready to bleed, then a point of dry ice is pressed on it for a few minutes, freezing it deeply. This treatment is repeated after a week or ten days, and after a similar interval a third treatment is given if needed. Cures are claimed in more than ninety per cent of the cases treated. In the case of soft warts paring is omitted, and these warts often disappear after only one freezing.

Found at Watering Places

The famous European spas which at one time were such favorite health resorts probably owed their beneficial effects to the fact that in most cases their waters were heavily charged with carbon dioxide. This made their waters slightly acid and greatly increased their mineral content. This was no doubt of great benefit to persons whose diet had been deficient in these minerals. Large quantities of the water were drunk in the effort to gain more benefit, and as a result devotees of the spas absorbed enough carbon dioxide from the water to quiet their nerves temporarily. This probably resulted in their taking a more relaxed attitude, both mentally and physically, so that they slept better and secured the adequate rest which may have been the primary need of many.

Probably the use of carbon dioxide with which the greatest number of people are familiar is in the production of carbonated drinks. This type of drink was originally called soda water, because the carbon dioxide in it was released from bicarbonate of soda (baking soda) as it combined with the acid in the drink. The original purpose was to produce an effervescent, sparkling, and tangy drink, but it seems more than possible that the originators of carbonated drinks had unknowingly stumbled upon an even more important sales appeal and business building quality. It is at least open to debate whether the great present-day popularity of various kinds of carbonated drinks is not due in some degree at least to the mildly sedative and relaxing effect of the carbon dioxide, which tends to give some relief to the tenseness of present-day life. That these drinks do have a definitely relaxing effect is proved by the fact that carbonated ginger ale is a very good remedy for hiccups, its effect probably being reinforced slightly by the holding of the breath during the process of drinking.

Little attention has been given to the possible connection between carbon dioxide and smoking. The smoke from tobacco, like smoke from the burning of any carbonaceous material, is composed largely of carbon dioxide. Because this gas passes so freely through all the body tissues, much of it is absorbed in the mouth and throat, even when the smoke is not inhaled. Consequently chain smokers tend to maintain an increased content of carbon dioxide in their blood almost continuously throughout their waking hours. The eventual effect of this is to develop a tolerance in the respiratory center of the brain so that it requires the increased carbon dioxide to maintain normal breathing. When smoking stops and carbon dioxide falls, breathing falls with it, resulting in an insufficient supply of oxygen to the lungs. This causes a feeling of uneasiness which the smoker relieves by smoking again. Dr. William Kaufman, of Bridgeport, Connecticut, in a letter to the Journal of the American Medical Society, suggests that smokers should relieve this feeling of uneasiness, not by having another smoke, but simply by giving conscious attention to their breathing and bringing it back to normal. Periods of normal breathing repeated frequently throughout the day will gradually restore the sensitiveness of the respiratory center. When this is accomplished, Dr. Kaufman says, smoking can be stopped with little difficulty.

If carbon dioxide is used in so many ways inside the body, what can be said about its uses outside the body? The answer is that they are almost unlimited. Here we can give only a few examples, but enough to illustrate the marvelous versatility of this gas. No list can be complete, because there are almost constant reports of still other uses that have been discovered or invented.

Used in Dry Ice

Great quantities of carbon dioxide are now used in the form of dry ice as a substitute for water ice in refrigeration. It has two great advantages over water ice. First, it will maintain a temperature more than a hundred degrees lower than water ice. Second, it changes directly from a solid to a gas and disappears into the air without leaving any residue behind, such as the water left by ordinary ice.

Probably the oldest and most universal man-made use of carbon dioxide is in the leavening of bread. Ancient peoples learned that permitting dough to ferment before baking produced a lighter, more porous bread. This fermentation was simply the growth of wild yeast plants which reached the dough through the air. These yeast plants, instead of using carbon dioxide in their growth to form starch and sugar, as most plants do, give off carbon dioxide as they make use of sugar and starch in their growth. The carbon dioxide which they produce is caught as bubbles in the dough, causing it to "rise." Most home baking still makes use of carbon dioxide, but now it is usually produced by baking powder, which gives the same effect as the earlier use of sour milk and soda. Both depend for their action on the carbon dioxide which is released from the "soda" (sodium bicarbonate) as it combines with the acid of the sour milk or the baking powder. In the baking powder the acid ingredient and the soda are mixed dry with some starch, so that no chemical reaction takes place between them until a liquid is added. This soda used in baking is identical with the sodium bicarbonate which plays such an important part in maintaining the acid-base balance of the blood. When the bread is eaten most of the carbon dioxide escapes into the air. The sodium is absorbed through the stomach and takes its normal part in the body's chemistry or is excreted as a surplus by the kidneys.

The preparation of sugar for our morning coffee requires the use of carbon dioxide in the refining process. Impurities in the raw juice from the beets or cane are removed by adding calcium hydrate (slaked lime). Then the lime must be removed from the juice. This is done by adding carbon dioxide, causing the lime to change its form to calcium carbonate (limestone), which is easily separated by settling and filtering. The juice having been cleared in this way is then evaporated under vacuum, the sugar crystallized, and the molasses separated in a centrifugal machine. Finally the sugar crystals are washed and dried and are ready for packing in the bags in which we buy them.

According to findings of the New York State Experiment Station, even the freshness of the eggs which we eat for breakfast depends largely on their content of carbon dioxide. Fresh eggs, it seems, are heavily charged with carbon dioxide, and unless some method is used to retain it, it escapes through the shell and is replaced by air, causing a rapid loss of freshness. Eggs that are immersed in water-glass (sodium silicate solution) or that have received a coating to prevent this loss of carbon dioxide have been found to retain their freshness over a much longer period. Professor Darrah of Cornell offers the suggestion that new-laid eggs should be removed from the shells and placed in plastic cups in which they could be charged with carbon dioxide and sealed to exclude air. Professor Darrah thinks the plastic cup would be a much better container than the shell the hen puts on the egg, being air-tight, break-proof, and transparent, and he would make the cups separable, so that the eggs could be boiled separately in the cups before they are opened. He says the sealed charge of carbon dioxide would keep the eggs fresh much longer, and he thinks housewives would prefer to see the eggs in the transparent cups rather than merely to see the shells when they are buying.

For Keeping Apples

Virginia Experiment Station researchers believe that with the aid of carbon dioxide they will be able in the near future to assure apple eaters a year-round supply of high quality dessert apples. At present apples are kept during the winter by maintaining them at a temperature not far above freezing. In this storage they are surrounded by ordinary air, which contains about twenty per cent of oxygen and only a fraction of one per cent of carbon dioxide. In the new method of storage the low temperature is still maintained, but nearly all the oxygen in the air of the storage room is removed and replaced with carbon dioxide. This change in the air delays the ripening process in the apples so much that it has increased the successful storage time as much as fifty per cent. Apples stored by this method also hold up longer after they are taken out of storage. Carbon dioxide storage is already widely used in England and on a more limited scale in New York and the New England states, especially for the McIntosh variety, which is excellent for eating but not a good keeper. With some further refinements it is expected that storage with carbon dioxide will soon be used widely with other favorite varieties, extending their marketing periods well into the summer.

This method of storage for apples is very similar to a method which has been used by the author of this book for several years past in preserving black walnut kernels. These kernels keep in perfect condition for years if left in their shells, but the shells are so hard that it is very inconvenient to crack the nuts as they are used. Consequently most of them are cracked where they are grown and only the kernels marketed. The kernels are very rich in oil which takes up oxygen from the air in warm weather and becomes rancid, giving the kernels an unpleasant flavor. In order to have pleasant-flavored kernels available in summer as well as winter the experiment was tried of keeping them in an atmosphere of carbon dioxide. Kernels sealed in the vapor from dry ice kept in perfect condition without refrigeration for a full year.

Just as its ability to prevent oxidation enables carbon dioxide to preserve the walnut kernels, the same characteristic makes it one of the most effective fire extinguishers. It is completely non-inflammable, and being heavier than air it tends to fall over and about any burning object and push away the air, thus preventing any further supply of oxygen from reaching the fire and making further burning impossible. It is especially valuable in oil and gasoline fires, because it is light enough to float on top of these substances, while water quickly sinks below them, leaving them still burning on top. When carbon dioxide is imprisoned as bubbles in a lather or foam, such as foamite, it forms a more permanent blanket which disperses into the air much more slowly and is therefore more effective.

Softens Up Oysters

One of the best proofs of the relaxing effect of carbon dioxide on muscles is found, surprisingly enough, not in a medical but in an industrial use of this gas. The shells of oysters are commonly held very tightly closed by a strong muscle inside the shell, so that considerable effort is required to open them. This causes delay and adds expense when oysters are being prepared for shipment or canning. Some years ago a specialist employed by the government was assigned to find ways to overcome this difficulty. He found that one of the most effective methods was simply to immerse the oysters in water containing a small percentage of carbon dioxide. In a short time this produced such a relaxation of the shell muscle that the shell could be opened easily.

What most people would consider an even more difficult task than opening an oyster's shell would be taking the pucker out of a persimmon. It had long been known that the Japanese had discovered a method by which they could remove the astringency from their native persimmons. So a government investigator was sent to Japan to find out what this method was. All he could learn was that the persimmons when harvested were always packed in empty sake kegs. Later when they were fully ripened and were taken out of the kegs the astringency was gone. He was assured that no other treatment had been given them. After considerable chemical detective work the secret was discovered. The wood of the kegs had become saturated with carbon dioxide from the fermenting sake, and when the sake was taken out and the kegs filled with persimmons the carbon dioxide escaped from the wood and penetrated the persimmons, evidently producing some chemical reaction inside them. Apparently no effort was made to determine what this chemical reaction was. On his return the investigator embodied his discoveries in a patent which he assigned to the U. S.

Government. Some years ago the author of this book by means of grafting grew some Chinese persimmons on his farm in Virginia. Chinese persimmons are more astringent than the Japanese. Even when left on the tree until they had been exposed to several frosts and were over-ripe, they were still unpleasant to eat. But after two or three months storage in an atmosphere of carbon dioxide all their astringency was gone and they were delightfully sweet.

According to a recent report carbon dioxide played an active part in Gulf Oil Company researches which resulted in the production of a special insecticide costing the company $18,000,000 a pound and considered worth the money. This valuable substance was a radioactive form of the widely used insect poison pyrethrum. The cost seems less prohibitive when we are told that only a thousandth part of a pound was made. To produce it pyrethrum plants were grown in a green house in air heavily charged with radioactive carbon dioxide. The radioactive carbon in this gas was taken up by the plants, which were then used to make the insecticide. By tracing the movement of the radioactive carbon in insects which have been poisoned by the pyrethrum the researchers expect to learn how the poison kills. Using this knowledge they hope to be able to develop a synthetic substitute for natural pyrethrum.

Slaughtering Made Easier

The statement has frequently been made that the big meat packers utilize every part of the hog except the squeal. This statement is no longer applicable to the more progressive packers, not because they have found a way to utilize the squeal, but because now there isn't any squeal. The pig passes into a compartment where the air contains a high percentage of carbon dioxide. Breathing this air he quickly falls into a deep surgical sleep. The conveyor then carries him past the butcher. But he does not feel the thrust of the knife which draws his life blood any more than a patient in a hospital feels the scalpel of the surgeon who operates on him. Now we can all eat our pork chops with a clearer conscience, knowing that through this merciful use of carbon dioxide the pig who contributed the chops was given a peaceful and painless passage from his earthly life. It has been found that a butcher can handle twice as many hogs in a day when they are under anesthesia and do it with less effort. Also the meat produced is of higher quality because the relaxed pig bleeds more freely and there is entire absence of the bruises commonly caused by his death struggles. A study by the U. S. Department of Agriculture has found that carbon dioxide can also be used successfully in slaughter houses for turkeys. The bruises and broken bones frequently caused by struggling birds no longer occur when the birds are quietly put to sleep before they are killed.

An ingenious use of carbon dioxide is in the filling of rigid air ships with helium. It is necessary that this operation be performed without any mixing of air with the helium. So the ship is first filled with carbon dioxide pumped in at the bottom. Being much heavier than air the carbon dioxide drives the air out at the top of the ship much as if the ship had been filled with water. Helium is then filled in from the top of the ship as the carbon dioxide is drawn off at the bottom. Because helium is so extremely light, there is very little mixing of the two gases, and only a small amount of helium has to be drawn off to clear the last of the carbon dioxide, and even this amount is not lost. Air and helium are very hard to separate, but carbon dioxide and helium are not. When the mixture is passed through a caustic solution the carbon dioxide is absorbed and the helium passes through unmixed. So in filling the ship by this method no helium is lost.

Probably few people know that the bell buoy at the entrance to Chesapeake Bay is operated by liquid carbon dioxide. A cylinder in the buoy is charged with 100 pounds of the liquid which discharges slowly as a gas and builds up pressure in an auxiliary cylinder. When this pressure approaches 300 pounds to the square inch it is released and drives a piston to produce a powerful stroke of the bell. The expansion of carbon dioxide in passing from the liquid form to a gas is so great that one load of the 100 pound cylinder provides power for 800,000 bell strokes.

Blasts Out Coal

The great expansive force of carbon dioxide in its liquid form is now being used in a number of coal mines to replace blasting powder and dynamite in blasting down coal. A two- or three-inch tube of strong alloy steel is loaded with liquid carbon dioxide and a chemical compound to furnish heat. For blasting, the tube is inserted in a drill hole in the coal vein and the heating compound ignited with a low voltage electric current. The inner end of the tube is closed with a thin steel disc which will rupture at any desired pressure from 10,000 to 20,000 pounds per square inch. Since liquid carbon dioxide boils at an extremely low temperature, very little heat is required to change it to the gaseous form. This builds up enormous pressure in the steel tube, ruptures the thin disc, and releases the carbon dioxide gas in a sudden explosive rush with the predetermined volume and pressure. Since the heat of the ordinary blast is absent, there is no danger of causing an explosion of coal dust or of accumulated seepage gas. In fact, the expanding carbon dioxide acts as a refrigerant, actually lowering the mine temperature. In addition the released carbon dioxide is a perfect fire extinguisher. Because of its safety, carbon dioxide blasting can be done throughout the working day instead of waiting until the miners are out of the mine. Also, since the violence of the explosions can be exactly controlled, it is possible to produce better coal, with a smaller percentage being shattered into dust.

Carbon dioxide has quickly found an important place even in the atomic age. When the British decided to build ten nuclear power plants over the ten-year period, 1955 to 1965 to reduce the drain on their dwindling coal supplies, one of the most important points they had to decide was what should be used as the coolant and heat transfer material in the reactors. After thorough study of the various available materials carbon dioxide was found to possess a combination of qualities which placed it at the head of the list. When Queen Elizabeth on Oct. 17, 1956, pulled the lever which turned electricity from the Calder Hall station into the nation's power lines England achieved the honor of possessing the world's first large-scale atomic power station. And in this station carbon dioxide was assigned the task of absorbing the fierce heat from the exploding atoms and carrying it to the boilers where steam is made to run the turbines of the electric generators.

An astonishing and almost incredible development in which carbon dioxide plays an essential part is the radiocarbon dating of past events through the remains of plants and animals. Bones, charcoal, wood, and other substances up to twenty thousand years old are made to tell their age within reasonably close limits by means of their content of radioactive carbon. Cosmic rays from outer space are constantly forming radioactive carbon dioxide in the air, maintaining it in a fairly constant proportion. Plants take up this radioactive carbon, and animals eat the plants, so that all plants and animals while they are alive have in them a uniform proportion of this active carbon. But at death they cease to take up fresh supplies, and that which they had accumulated disintegrates at a steady rate, as all radioactive substances do. At the end of 5,760 years half of this radioactive carbon will have been lost, and after 5,760 more years only one-fourth of the original amount will remain. So from the amount of radioactive carbon which remains in any animal or vegetable substance its age can be calculated.

CO_2 Affects Our Climate

As if carbon dioxide were not already known to affect our lives in enough different ways, a Johns Hopkins physicist now comes forward with figures to show that this gas plays a large part in determining our climate. Recent calculations he has made show that carbon dioxide is much more opaque to long-wave heat radiation than had previously been supposed. This means that the carbon dioxide distributed through the atmosphere acts like the glass in a greenhouse. It allows the short-wave heat from the ten-thousand degree surface of the sun to come through and warm the earth, but at the same time it prevents the low-temperature long-wave heat of the earth from escaping, as it otherwise would, by radiation into space. This results in a much greater accumulation of the sun's heat on the earth and consequently a warmer climate. In the near future a perceptible warming up of our climate may result from the burning of coal, oil, and other carbonaceous fuels on the vast scale demanded by modern industry. Scientists calculate that in the next fifty years one and three-quarters billion tons of carbon dioxide will be added to the earth's atmosphere. As a result Russia, which is now almost wholly landlocked, may in fifty years become a great merchant-marine power. Fantastic as it sounds, scientists believe that carbon dioxide gas given off from burning fuels may retain the sun's heat and warm up Russia's Arctic coastline sufficiently to make its ports ice-free for all or most of the year.

It seems likely that in the near future carbon dioxide will be called upon to give an extra boost to the production of food for the world's rapidly increasing population. The Carnegie Institution has begun investigation into the large-scale growth of improved types of seaweeds known as algae. These plants contain a very high percentage of protein, and their growth has been found to be most rapid when they are grown in air which has had its natural content of carbon dioxide considerably increased. It is estimated that if grown under the most favorable conditions algae could produce on an area twice the size of Rhode Island enough protein to meet the full requirement of the entire present population of the earth. A highly improved strain of algae stimulated by flashes of intense light gives promise of supplying substantial amounts of food and oxygen for submariners, and eventually for space men, even when grown in their limited quarters.

Comes from Limestone

Since carbon dioxide is used for so many purposes the question may arise as to where so much of it comes from or how it is produced commercially. Most of it comes from heating limestone. At a temperature of seven or eight hundred degrees the limestone separates into carbon dioxide, water, and calcium oxide, or quicklime. The calcium oxide remains as a solid residue, and the carbon dioxide comes off as a gas mixed with water in the form of steam. When this mixture is cooled the water separates as liquid leaving practically pure carbon dioxide which can be easily collected in large quantities. The residual quicklime has many industrial uses and its sale covers a large part of the expense of producing the carbon dioxide, making it a relatively inexpensive gas. Of course there are great quantities of carbon dioxide in the air, but in comparison with the vast total volume of the air its amount is very small, only about three one-hundredths of one per cent, so that the cost of separating it from the air would be prohibitive. Natural gas as it comes from the well contains a considerable percentage of carbon dioxide. Since it can combine with no additional oxygen and so can take no part in the burning of the remainder of the gas, its presence merely serves to reduce the heat of the flame and to lower the heating value of the gas. At least one company has found it profitable to improve its gas by separating the carbon dioxide, which is then sold as dry ice. Recently a method of producing carbon dioxide by burning petroleum gases in oxygen has been developed which promises to be commercially practicable.

Amazing as are the varied uses of carbon dioxide sketched in this chapter, its use in promoting sleep is no less amazing. In fact, the victim of insomnia who masters its use will probably consider its sleep-producing power the most amazing of all.